ANTIBIOTICS AND
ANTIBIOTIC RESISTANCE

This book is du⸱⸱

ANTIBIOTICS AND ANTIBIOTIC RESISTANCE

Ola Sköld, M.D., Ph.D.
Professor of Microbiology
Uppsala University

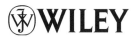

A JOHN WILEY & SONS, INC., PUBLICATION

Published by John Wiley & Sons, Inc., Hoboken, New Jersey
Published simultaneously in Canada

For general information on our other products and services or for technical support, please contact our Customer Care Department within the United States at (800) 762-2974, outside the United States at (317) 572-3993 or fax (317) 572-4002.

Wiley also publishes its books in a variety of electronic formats. Some content that appears in print may not be available in electronic formats. For more information about Wiley products, visit our web site at www.wiley.com.

Library of Congress Cataloging-in-Publication Data:

Sköld, Ola.
  [Antibiotika och antibiotikaresistens. English]
  Antibiotics and antibiotic resistance / Ola Sköld.
    p. ; cm.
  Translation of: Antibiotika och antibiotikaresistens / Ola Sköld. c2006.
  Includes index.
  ISBN 978-0-470-43850-3 (cloth)
 1. Antibiotics. 2. Drug resistance in microorganisms. I. Title.
  [DNLM: 1. Anti-Bacterial Agents. 2. Drug Resistance, Microbial. QV 350]
  RM267.S55513 2011
  615'.329–dc22

                          2011002200

Printed in the United States of America

ePDF ISBN: 978-1-118-07556-2
oBook ISBN: 978-1-118-07560-9
ePub ISBN: 978-1-118-07558-6

10 9 8 7 6 5 4 3 2 1

To the memory of J. B. Neilands, Professor of Biochemistry,
University of California, Berkeley
"The finest Gentleman of Science I ever met"

CONTENTS

4 PENICILLINS AND OTHER BETALACTAMS   69

5 GLYCOPEPTIDES   95

PREFACE

By controlling bacterial infections, antibiotics have given us a health standard that we have become used to and which would be very difficult to lose. Antibiotics are unique among medicines in that they act selectively on bacteria, among them the pathogens, while leaving human cells and tissues unaffected. A description of how antibiotics work and of the mechanisms by which bacteria resist them often falls between the medical discipline of infectious diseases and the field of microbiology. With this book I mean to bridge this gap. It should serve as a brief handbook for physicians, veterinarians, and pharmacists and as a textbook for students in these areas of study. I also describe the rapid and very worrying development of antibiotic resistance among pathogenic bacteria, including the molecular mechanisms of this resistance and newly observed genetic principles for the spread of resistance among species.

Our ubiquitous use of antibiotics for medical purposes and for growth promotion in farm animals has been a toxic shock to the microbial world, which has responded by developing resistance. It can be looked upon as a piece of Darwinian evolution taking place right in front of us. Genes mediating resistance, mostly of unknown origin, have been shown to be spread by means of earlier unknown and very efficient genetic mechanisms. No microbiologist can escape being astonished and impressed by the ingenuity of evolution in finding and combining molecular mechanisms to protect the bacterial world from the dramatic environmental change that our use of antibiotics has effected.

Finally, I describe the future possibilities that, under the threat of resistance evolution, can be envisioned to help maintain the health standard that antibiotics have helped us reach in controlling bacterial infections, which we have come to take for granted.

Ola Sköld, M.D., Ph.D.

CHAPTER 1

ANTIBIOTICS: THE GREATEST TRIUMPH OF SCIENTIFIC MEDICINE

The use of antibiotics has given us medical control of bacterial infections. This is a health standard that we have become accustomed to and have come to regard as self-evident. Today, it is impossible to imagine health care that is not able to cope efficiently with bacterial infections. Medical disciplines such as oncology and organ transplantation surgery would simply collapse without access to modern antibiotics.

The tremendous success of antibiotics in the field of infectious diseases for seven decades or so has led to very wide distribution and consumption of these agents. Besides their medical use for human beings and animals, antibiotics have been used in very large quantities as growth stimulants in husbandry and as prophylactic protection against plant pathogens. All this has led to the spread of millions of tons of antibiotics in the biosphere during the antibiotics epoch. This has induced a drastic environmental change, a toxic shock to the bacterial world. It has been said that "the world is immersed in a dilute solution of antibiotics."

Antibiotics and Antibiotics Resistance, First Edition. Ola Sköld.
© 2011 John Wiley & Sons, Inc. Published 2011 by John Wiley & Sons, Inc.

Bacteria have adjusted to the changed environment in the usual method used by living organisms: by evolution. The bacterial world, including human pathogens, has developed and mobilized molecular defense mechanisms for protection against the human-produced poisons that antibiotics are. This has led to increased antibiotics resistance among human pathogens, which are becoming more difficult to treat. This poses a serious threat to our health standard in that the ability of medicine to cope with bacterial infections has slowly been eroded. Medical journals and daily newspapers report on cases of infectious disease that were untreatable because of antibiotics resistance. One recent report described a young woman dying of tuberculosis despite intensive treatment. The tuberculosis bacteria causing the disease were multiply resistant and thus resisted treatment with all available antituberculosis drugs. What is happening, and what is going to happen?

Harmful cells comprise the two greatest threats to our health. In the first case, our own cells lose their growth regulation by genetic changes, thereby causing cancer. In the second, foreign organisms infect and establish themselves in the tissues of the human body, inhibiting their functions and destroying them by the action of toxins. Bacteria form the dominant part of the latter group: tuberculosis, syphilis, cholera, typhus, typhoid fever, and bubonic plague, for example. The medical treatment of cancer and that of bacterial infections are related in that both include the use of cell growth–inhibiting or cell-killing agents. Cancer cells are treated with cytostatics, which are difficult to use and must be handled by oncology specialists. This is because cancer cells originate from normal cells and are metabolically very similar to normal cells, letting cytostatics also interfere with healthy cells, such as those of the bone marrow, where the continuous growth of cells is necessary for the support of life.

SELECTIVITY

Bacteria belong to another biological world and are structurally and metabolically very different from our cells. They can be inhibited in growth and also killed by agents that do not interfere with our cells. That is, antibacterial agents, antibiotics, used for clinical purposes in medicine must act selectively on bacteria. Their handling can therefore be focused on the characteristics of the infecting bacterium.

Penicillin was discovered more than 80 years ago. Penicillin and its many followers, all with a selectively inhibiting effect on bacteria, had a tremendous impact on the treatment of infectious diseases and on their panorama of occurrence in the first decades of their ubiquitous clinical use (1950–1980). The great clinical success of antibiotics changed the attitude of the medical profession toward bacterial infections. This is reflected in a statement from 1969 by the Surgeon General, William H. Stewart, to the U.S. Congress: "It is time to close the book on infectious diseases." The surgeon general is the highest medical officer in the U.S. Department of Health and Human Services.

Antibiotics are unique among pharmaceutical remedies in that they do not direct their action toward our own cells but selectively toward foreign cells, bacteria coming from the outside and infecting our tissues. Their selective action means that they must target physiological and biochemical differences between our cells and bacterial cells in order to effect bacteriostatic or bacteriocidal activity. The key property of clinically useful antibacterial agents, then, is selectivity. It can be noted that in the search for new antibiotics in molds and other microorganisms, with *Penicillium* as an example, many selective and useful antibiotics were found (e.g., streptomycin and rifampicin), but also others with a good antibacterial effect but without selectivity, making them unusable for the clinical treatment of bacterial infections. The latter antibiotics show inhibiting or killing activity toward both bacteria and our cells, and have in some cases (e.g., adriamycin, bleomycin, and mitomycin) found use as cytostatic agents in the treatment of cancer, and then under the usual strict oncologist control of, among other things, bone marrow function.

DEVELOPMENT OF RESISTANCE

Since antibiotics are only active against foreign cells, bacteria, and should have no effect on our cells and tissues, they are not pharmacologically active, except for side effects that occur with several of them when given in large doses. This means that they can be prescribed less strictly than other pharmaceuticals. In many patients showing signs of infection they are given simply for safety, without a strict bacterial diagnosis. This has contributed heavily to the very large consumption of antibiotics that can be estimated from sales figures, which can be used as good proxies for actual consumption (Chapter 2).

Resistance to antibiotics among pathogenic bacteria has developed within a short time and in many ways faster than could have been expected. This can be explained partially by the short generation time of bacteria, allowing them to undergo a Darwinian evolution in a much shorter time than has been possible for animals and other organisms. Furthermore, bacteria have the ability to manipulate their own genetic makeup, leading to a faster adaptation to the toxic effects of antibiotics: that is, the development of resistance. It can be looked upon as the natural genetic engineering of bacteria, including the uptake and incorporation of resistance-mediating genes from related organisms by adaptation of evolutionary old genetic mechanisms to the new environmental situation of the large presence of antibiotics. No microbiologist can escape feeling surprise and wonder as these phenomena continuously unfold.

Resistance is the dark and daunting side of the antibiotics triumph, and we are forced to realize that the health standard that antibiotics have given us is not stable. The great asset that antibiotics represent is devalued by the evolution of resistance. In a longer perspective this development is quite threatening. Many medical specialities are dependent on efficient antibiotics. Will we be able to maintain control of bacterial infections, or will our descendants look back nostalgically and talk about the time that we had both oil and antibiotics?

SULFONAMIDE: THE FIRST ANTIBACTERIAL AGENT ACTING SELECTIVELY

Louis Pasteur, a great French microbiologist of the nineteenth century, formulated and proposed what was called the *germ theory of disease*, the concept that infectious disease was caused by microorganisms. Later, Robert Koch at the Imperial Health Office in Berlin provided proof, with *Bacillus antracis* as an example, that there is a definite causal relation of a particular microorganism to a particular disease. From these ideas Koch formulated his postulates for characterizing a pathogenic microbe:

1. The organism is found regularly in the lesions of the disease.
2. It can be isolated in pure culture on artificial media.
3. Inoculation of this culture produces the disease in experimental animals.
4. The organism can be recovered from lesions in these animals.

Based on these basic ideas, Paul Ehrlich at the Royal Institute for Experimental Therapy in Frankfurt am Main advanced the idea of direct selective action of a drug on infecting microbes. His expression for this was the "magic bullet," which would exhibit a greater affinity for pathogenic bacteria than for host cells. For this selective action he coined the word *chemotherapy*. Ehrlich further observed that dyes stained different cell components selectively and proposed the idea that organic stains taken up, particularly by living cells, could have a therapeutic effect by interfering with bacterial infections.

In the 1930s, these ideas led Gerhard Domagk, who was working at the Institute of Experimental Pathology at the I.G. Farbenindustrie in Elberfeld, Germany, to the discovery of Prontosil rubrum (4-sulfonamide-2',4'-diaminoazobenzol, Domagk 1935) (Fig. 1.1); a chemically synthesized dye of red color, which showed an effect against bacterial infections in animals. It was, however, inactive in vitro. Jaques and Therese Tréfouël of the Pasteur Institute in France could show that patients treated with Prontosil excreted a simpler product, sulfanilamide, which was active in vivo as well as in vitro against the growth of bacteria. This was a dramatic development since it finally established Ehrlich's principle of chemotherapeutic action. Sulfanilamide is a colorless substance and not a dye, partly contradicting the theory leading to its discovery.

Sulfanilamide was set free from the dye by hydrolysis in vivo in animal experiments. Sulfanilamide was thus the first antibacterial agent to act selectively. The first trials of Prontosil rubrum on animals were performed by Domagk in 1932. He could show that mice infected experimentally with *Streptococcus pyogenes* by injection into the peritoneum were protected from peritonitis with this agent. The results were published in *Deutsche medizinische Wochenschrift* in 1935, and sulfonamides were soon used widely for the clinical treatment of infections with streptococci, staphylococci, meningococci, and other severely pathogenic bacterial agents. Domagk's work is unjustly forgotten today but was much appreciated by his contemporaries, and at the end of

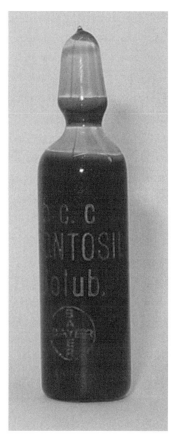

FIGURE 1.1 Sulfonamide. Ampoule containing 5 mL of Prontosil rubrum for injection, the first sulfonamide preparation for clinical use.

the 1930s he was nominated for the Nobel Prize in Physiology or Medicine. The Nazi regime of that time in Germany had, however, declared that it did not want to see any German as a Nobel laureate, probably because of the Nobel committee's choice of earlier Nobel Peace Prize laureates. The German government of that time tried through its embassy in Stockholm, and also directly through the foreign office in Berlin, to interfere with the work of the Nobel committee at the Karolinska Institute in

Stockholm. The Nobel committee, with its chairman pathology professor Folke Henschen, stood up to the pressure, however, and asked the medical faculty at the Karolinska Institute to award the prize to Domagk. In his memoirs from 1957, Folke Henschen, who personally knew Gerhard Domagk, mentioned that in the night following that day in October 1939 when the prize was announced, Domagk was arrested by Nazi soldiers in his home in Wuppertal and taken to jail. Next morning, when the prison director made his daily round, he met with Domagk, who did not seem to fit the environment. "Who are you?" he asked. "I am Professor Gerhard Domagk of the University of Münster." *"Weshalb sind Sie hier denn?"* Domagk's reply: *"Ich habe den Nobel-preis bekommen."* The Nazi authorities did not allow Domagk to travel to Stockholm to receive the prize in December 1939. He did not go to Stockholm to receive the medal and the diploma until 1947, but because Alfred Nobel's will specifies that the offer of prize money expires on the day of the award ceremony, he received no prize money.

Sulfonamides chemically synthesized beginning with Domagk's Prontosil rubrum were widely used as efficient and inexpensive antibacterial drugs for the treatment of both gram-positive and gram-negative pathogens, and they had a deep impact on the fate of Europe. In December 1943, British Prime Minister Winston Churchill had just completed a complex series of meetings, among them the fateful conference with Franklin D. Roosevelt and the Soviet leader Joseph V. Stalin in Teheran. He was on his way to meet with the U.S. General Dwight D. Eisenhower in Tunis to discuss the D-day landings when he contracted a severe case of pneumonia. His doctor, Lord Moran, decided to treat his important patient with a new drug, a sulfonamide. The treatment was successful, and there is little doubt that the novel sulfa drug defeated the pneumonia and probably saved the life of this important European leader.

Chemotherapeutics and Antibiotics

The chemically synthesized sulfonamide was the first antibacterial agent to act selectively. The introduction of sulfonamide into clinical practice can be regarded as the birth of chemotherapy as defined by Paul Ehrlich. Through the years, however, the term *chemotherapy* has come to mean treatment with cytostatic agents in the treatment of tumors. The original distinction between chemotherapeutics, chemically synthesized antibacterial agents such as sulfonamides, and antibiotics produced by living organisms has been difficult to retain, not least because medicinal chemists have been increasingly skillful in modifying antibiotic structures: for example, to escape resistance development (Chapter 4). The term *chemotherapeutics* is not used much at present. Instead, the word *antibiotics* has come to comprise all selectively acting antibacterial agents, even though the meaning of the word is not altogether correct when applied to antibacterial agents such as sulfonamides, trimethoprim, and linezolide.

PENICILLIN: THE FIRST ANTIBIOTIC

Penicillin was the first antibiotic in the strict sense of the word: that is, an antibacterial agent produced in a living organism. The original observation was made by Alexander Fleming at the bacteriological laboratory of Saint Mary's Hospital in London. In his research, Fleming was interested in staphylococci, particularly in the color and form of staphylococcal colonies on an agar plate. He had a hypothesis, which could never be verified, that there was a connection between the appearance of staphylococcal colonies and their pathogenicity. Among his staphylococcal plates, on one occasion, Fleming observed a plate with a large patch of mold growing on it (Fig. 1.2). The staphylococcal colonies on the same plate seemed to maintain a distance from the mold, not growing in its vicinity.

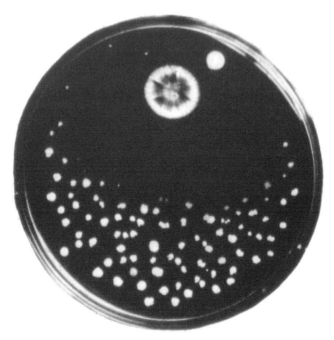

FIGURE 1.2 The discovery of penicillin. A replica of the original plate of Alexander Fleming showing a patch of *Penicillium* mold and *Staphylococcus* colonies seeming to avoid the mold patch.

This phenomenon caught Fleming's attention, and one of the many biographies about him (Gwyn Macfarlane, *Alexander Fleming, The Man and the Myth*, The Hogarth Press, London, 1984) describes how on a sunny September morning in 1928 on the lawn outside the laboratory, he showed the plate to two fellow bacteriologists. None of the three could explain the phenomenon on the plate or at all imagine that at that moment they had a tryst with destiny. The interpretation of this phenomenon would open the way for the greatest triumph of scientific medicine: the control of bacterial infections with selectively acting drugs. The full impact of the observation was finally appreciated, and the original agar plate, showing antagonism between two microorganisms via a soluble agent, is now in the British Museum in

London. The diffusible agent inhibiting bacterial growth on the plate in the vicinity of the mold was named *penicillin* by Fleming, and together with its many derivatives, it would eventually become dominant among antibiotics in the treatment of bacterial disease.

There is another whim of destiny in the penicillin story. By its mechanism of action (Chapter 4), penicillin cannot act on resting nondividing bacterial cells—only on growing bacteria. This circumstance, together with the property of mold to grow much more slowly than staphylococci, led to the conclusion that penicillin could not have been discovered in the manner described. If the agar plate was already polluted with mold cells when Fleming streaked it with the staphylococci he was interested in, they would have grown out to be insusceptible to penincillin long before the mold had grown out enough to produce penicillin. The mold could also not have grown out to form a colony before inoculation with bacteria, since no microbiologist would use a contaminated agar plate. This microbiological mystery seems to be explained by a fantastic sequence of coincident circumstances. Fleming seems to have inoculated the agar plate at the end of the month of July and then left for summer holiday in Scotland, forgetting that the plate was on the bench and thus not placed in the 37°C incubator. The weather records for London from 1928 show that the first week of August that year was unusually cold, followed by hot summer weather. Mold cells grow faster than bacteria at low temperatures, which means that a mold colony could have formed during the cold spell, while the staphylococci caught up in the following warm period, then to meet with the penicillin produced and diffused out from the mold, forming the famous zone. This could be looked at as an example of *serendipity*, a scientist finding something quite significant without having looked for it (Fig. 1.3).

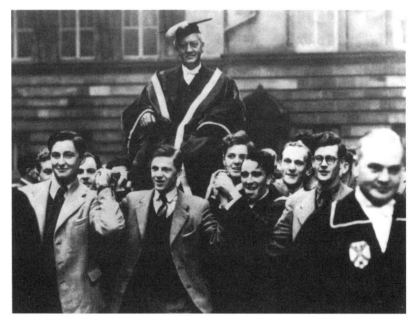

FIGURE 1.3   Sir Alexander Fleming celebrated by students at the University of Edinburgh.

The First Therapeutic Trial

Fleming identified the penicillin-producing mold as *Penicillium notatum* and showed that extracts from cultures of it inhibited the growth of several pathogenic bacterial strains. He also studied toxicity and therapeutic possibilities in animal experiments. Fleming left this research after about half a year, however, with a report delivered on May 10, 1929 and published in the June issue of *British Journal of Experimental Pathology* (No 3, volume 40). In this paper the therapeutic possibilities of penicillin are only mentioned in connection with the treatment of infected wounds. It is an enigma in the history of medicine why Fleming left research on penicillin so quickly. The most important reason for that was probably his observation that injected penicillin disappeared from the circulating blood of a rabbit within half an hour, whereas test tube experiments needed longer to show the growth-inhibiting effect on bacteria. Fleming's basic observations on penicillin were developed further toward an antibacterial remedy only after a period of 12 years, in 1940.

Rediscovery of Penicillin by a Basic Scientific Approach

In 1940, Australian-born Howard Florey, a professor of pathology, German-born Ernst Chain, a biochemist, and British-born Norman Heatley, a biochemist, all three at Oxford, England, began scientific studies on penicillin. Fleming had shown that penicillin interfered with the bacterial cell wall, and the three men wanted to investigate agents that had the ability to dissolve the murein of the cell wall in parallel with the enzyme lysozyme, the mechanism of action of which Florey had just studied. Chain first thought of penicillin as an enzyme, but very soon during purification, it emerged as a small molecule. After further purification the therapeutic possibilities could be discerned. It is interesting to note that it was purely a scientific interest in bacterial cell wall degradation that led the three scientists to take up study of the phenomenon discovered by Fleming. The realization of therapeutic possibilities led to what has been called the most important pharmaceutical experiment ever carried out. It began on Saturday morning, May 25, 1940, in Oxford when Howard Florey injected eight laboratory mice intraperitoneally, each with 10^8 cells of S. pyogenes. One hour later, four of the eight mice were injected subcutaneously with 10 mg of a brown powder dissolved in water. At half past three on Sunday morning, all four of the mice injected with the brown powder solution were healthy and agile, whereas the other four were dead. The brown powder was penicillin, but only 0.1% of it was actually penicillin; 99.9% constituted impurities.

The experiment indicated that penicillin could be developed into an important medicine, and Florey and Chain, in collaboration with Norman Heatley, tried to solve the biggest problem at the time: to grow *P. notatum* in sufficient volume to be able to purify penicillin from the growth medium in medically usable quantities. Heatley was the co-worker who devised a purification method and also the method needed to assay penicillin activity. The resources of Oxford were limited because of World War II, but with help from the American pharmaceutical industry, production was begun. The penicillin produced quickly performed as a dramatically efficient remedy against bacterial infections. It immediately provided great relief in the treatment of infected war wounds, and very soon it found its way into clinical medicine in general. Alexander Fleming, Howard Florey, and Ernst Chain were awarded the Nobel Prize in Physiology or Medicine in 1945. Today, penicillin is produced in copious amounts all over the world using industrial procedures that are so efficient that the final product is pure enough for direct use in pharmaceutical products. The large global production of penicillin today has led to it being regarded as a commodity on the scale of coffee and tea. Organic chemists have succeeded in the total synthesis of penicillin, but industrial production today takes place in large tanks where penicillin-producing mold cells are grown. The original *P. notatum* has been replaced by *Penicillium chrysogenum*, which is a more efficient producer.

Betalactams

The penicillin isolated originally, penicillin G, is acid labile and has to be administered parenterally lest it be destroyed by stomach acid. One of the first important derivatives of penicillin G was phenoxymethylpenicillin (penicillin V), which is acid stable and can be given by mouth. The characterization

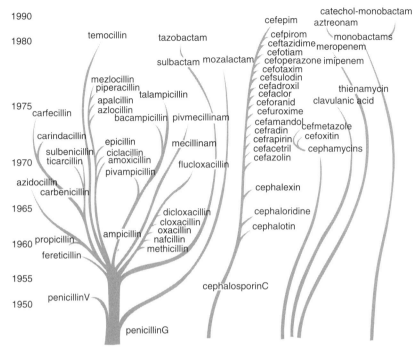

FIGURE 1.4   Overview of betalactams (see also Chapter 4). The left part of the figure depicts the relationships among betalactams as a tree with its roots in the penicillin-producing mold *Penicillium chrysogenum*. The clinical introduction of the various derivatives is given approximately by the time scale to the left.

of the betalactam ring of penicillin as the active component of the molecule has extended this group of antibiotics to a large family, the betalactams, including penicillins, cephalosporins, and monobactams (see also Chapter 4 and Fig. 1.4). The incitement for finding all these betalactams has been both to find antibacterials against pathogens with varying susceptibilities to betalactams, and to counteract the development of resistance (see also Chapter 4).

STREPTOMYCIN: THE SECOND ANTIBIOTIC IN THE HISTORY OF ANTIBACTERIAL AGENTS

The tremendous success of penicillin as an antibacterial agent isolated from a living organism induced an intensive search for further antibiotics among other microorganisms. Selman Waksman at Rutgers University was a well-known expert on soil microbes at the time (Fig. 1.5). Waksman was particularly interested in the antagonism between microorganisms as a means to understanding how soil microbes interact. It was said that one morning around 1940 he exclaimed to his collaborators: "Stop

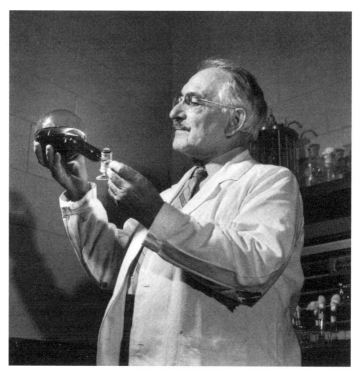

FIGURE 1.5 Selman Waksman, discoverer of streptomycin. In this photograph note the burn hole in the elbow of the lab coat, which is often characteristic of microbiologists, caused by the small, easily overlooked ignition flame of a bunsen burner.

what you are doing. Look at what those English can do with a mold. I know that organisms in the soil can do a lot more—let's start looking." Waksman's laboratory, among others, started the search for antibacterial agents among soil microorganisms. He and his co-workers concentrated their search on *Actinomyces* species and very soon found the two antibacterials actinomycin and streptothricin, which were, however, too toxic for use as antibacterial remedies. Actinomycin was toxic because it did not act selectively. Later it was put to good use as a cytostatic agent in the treatment of certain fast-growing forms of cancer, such as the epithelioma of the chorion, and streptothricin has been used for veterinary purposes in some parts of the world.

Further research by the group at Rutgers University resulted in the finding of streptomycin, which has been regarded as the second great antibiotic after penicillin. It had a dramatic medical impact because it was the first effective agent against *Mycobacterium tuberculosis* and thus the first effective remedy for tuberculosis, against which penicillin is not effective. The discovery was published in 1944 in *Proceedings of the Society for Experimental Biology and Medicine* in a paper, "Streptomycin: a Substance Exhibiting Antibiotic Activity Against Gram Positive and Gram Negative Bacteria." The first author of the paper was Albert Schatz, a graduate student of Waksman's. He had isolated one of the streptomycin-producing strains of *Streptomyces griseus* and also tested the effect of this new antibiotic on different bacteria. He would, however, not have been able to do this without access to the expertise on soil microorganisms and the system of methods available in Waksman's laboratory. The discovery of streptomycin was not at the time regarded as anything genuinely new in the scientific world, but as a development of concepts formulated in the breakthrough of penicillin as a medicine. Streptomycin won fame, however, as the first remedy against tuberculosis, and Waksman was awarded the

Nobel Prize in Medicine or Physiology in 1952. It was awarded to Waksman alone. Although Albert Schatz was responsible for the actual discovery, he was not included in the prize. This and the substantial amounts of royalty money that the commercial distribution of streptomycin as a pharmaceutical would bring in led to one of the bitterest feuds the world of science has ever seen. It continued for more than two decades, and included lawsuits, most of which Waksman won.

The protocols and regulations of the Nobel Committee at the Karolinska Institute are kept confidential for 50 years, so those regarding Waksman are now accessible for scrutiny. The streptomycin discovery, particularly with reference to the treatment of tuberculosis, was the subject of several reports and evaluations at that time. The most important one was dated August 21, 1952, and was signed by Einar Hammarsten, then professor and head of the Department of Medical and Physiological Chemistry at the Karolinska Institute. Hammarsten expressed himself very clearly, specifying that the discovery of streptomycin belonged to Waksman alone. He argued that the first streptomycin-producing strain of *S. griseus* was isolated by Waksman and that he had worked out the procedure for the isolation of streptothricin, which was also used for the original purification of streptomycin. The most important early publications on streptomycin carry many young authors' names, including Albert Schatz, Elisabeth Bugie, and Boyd Woodruff. Hammarsten wrote that these young co-workers could not be included as prizewinners.

The First Remedy for Tuberculosis

Streptomycin was the first efficient remedy against tuberculosis, and it quickly reduced mortality from this disease. It soon turned out, however, that it had severe clinical side effects. The most important were toxic effects on the sensory cells in the cochlea and vestibulum, in many cases leading to deafness and to interference with body balance. The precise toxic effect of streptomycin is directed toward the sensory cells registering the pressure changes of sound, and seems to be mediated by its binding to the melanin in cochlea. Nowadays these clinical problems with side effects can be handled by using drug combinations and by carefully following the serum concentrations of the drug in combination with close observations of hearing ability.

CONCLUSION

Sulfonamide, penicillin, and streptomycin were the harbingers of the antibiotics era. The promises of these agents regarding effective control of all types of bacterial disease have largely been fulfilled by the broad array of antibacterial agents now available. Today, it is difficult to imagine the fear and anxiety connected to the earlier panorama of infectious disease. There is evidence from world literature: for example, a famous novel from 1924, *Magic Mountain* by Thomas Mann, later earning its author the Nobel Prize in Literature. In that great novel there is a description of the relentless progress of tuberculosis despite many, often very painful treatments given the patients at Berghof, a rather luxurious sanatorium in the Swiss Alps. The description is frightening and fearful to us today, who feel relief at an x-ray diagnosis of tuberculosis—because the aberrant structure seen on the screen is not cancer. Tuberculostatic agents promise healing within months, and in the Western world, the number of deaths in tuberculosis has decreased about 1000-fold since 1900.

Is it possible to come to grips with antibiotics resistance, or are we on our way back to an inability to handle pathogenic bacteria? In actuality there is no real reason for fear. Most bacterial infections can still be treated efficiently, but there are many serious difficulties on the horizon.

CHAPTER **2**

DISTRIBUTION
OF ANTIBIOTICS

There is a direct correlation between the distribution of antibiotics and the development of resistance, in that ubiquitous spread of antibiotics makes resistance a survival condition for bacteria. Resistant bacteria are selected to grow and spread. If quantitative data on the distribution of antibiotics can be acquired, the pressure for selection of resistant bacteria and the risk of resistance development could be evaluated. Local and international figures for comparisons of antibiotics distribution are important in organizational efforts to curb resistance-inducing overconsumption of antibiotics, and in that way to lower the selection pressure for resistant bacteria and delay the development of resistance. The annual use of antimicrobials in the United States is large. Figures show that about 1500 metric tons are distributed each year for therapeutic and prophylactic human use. About the same quantity is distributed for therapeutic use in animals, and about 7400 metric tons are distributed for nontherapeutic (i.e., growth-promoting) purposes in animal husbandry.

Antibiotics and Antibiotics Resistance, First Edition. Ola Sköld.
© 2011 John Wiley & Sons, Inc. Published 2011 by John Wiley & Sons, Inc.

QUANTITATIVE EVALUATION OF ANTIBIOTICS CONSUMPTION

The development of resistance is related to the selection pressure of distributed antibiotics. Is it possible to measure this pressure quantitatively? Sales figures have been found to be a good proxy for true consumption. If sales and distribution are expressed in defined daily doses, the amounts of consumption become truly comparable between time periods and, for example, between different hospitals and different geographical areas. This approach will also reveal trends in the use of antibiotics.

Defined Daily Doses

A defined daily dose (DDD) is an international unit that expresses the recommended average dose per day for adults for treatment of the principal target for the pharmaceutical agent (for DDD values of various pharmaceuticals, see www.whocc.no). Numbers of DDD per 1000 inhabitants per day reflect the exposure of a population to a pharmaceutical agent. A distribution value of 20 DDD per 1000 inhabitants per day could, for example, be roughly translated into the exposure of 2% of the population for the agent in question.

International Distribution of Antibiotics:
A Scandinavian Example

Figures based on sales for the quantitative distribution of antibiotics reached a peak in Sweden in 1993: 19.4 DDD per 1000 inhabitants per day. This corresponds to 64 million defined daily doses for the entire population that year, which in turn corresponds to one week of antibiotics treatment for every Swede that year. In later years antibiotics consumption decreased slowly by about 30%, down to 14 DDD per 1000 inhabitants per day; it has fluctuated slightly with small increases for some years. There is also a substantial difference in antibiotics consumption between different parts of the country. In the sparsely populated northern areas, antibiotics consumption is just about 70% of that seen in the more densely populated southern areas. In the top year, 1993, a northern county showed an antibiotics consumption of 16.7 DDD per 1000 inhabitants per day, whereas the southern-most county showed a corresponding figure of 23.8 DDD per 1000 inhabitants per day. Taken into account that the Swedish population is relatively homogeneous, these large differences cannot reflect differences in the infection panorama but must be related to variations in prescription patterns for many non-medical reasons. Further analysis of these reasons ought to be useful in efforts to curb the overconsumption of antibiotics in general.

Similar differences in the consumption of antibiotics can also be observed in hospitals, where typically, 30 to 60% of inpatients are treated with antibiotics. The total consumption expressed as DDD per 1000 hospital days could vary twofold between large hospitals and also among those with a university affiliation. As specific examples, the consumption of tetracyclines could vary sixfold and cephalosporins almost fourfold between hospitals. These differences imply overconsumption and are so large that they could not be explained by differences in the panorama of infectious diseases, given that all the hospitals investigated included clinics for infectious diseases.

International comparisons also give the impression that antibiotics are overconsumed. A comparison of antibiotics consumption among the Nordic countries of Finland, Sweden, Norway, Iceland, and Denmark showed, for example, that the consumption expressed as DDD per 1000 inhabitants per day in Finland and Iceland is 25% larger than that in Sweden, while Norway shows about 10% lower values, and Denmark at least 17 to 18% lower values. Despite very homogeneous and similar populations with a very similar range of infectious diseases, there are thus considerable differences in antibiotics consumption among the Nordic countries. A comparison between Canada (British Columbia) and the European average showed that the Canadian consumption of antibiotics was comparable to that in Sweden but that the European average was more than 10% higher. Data on antibiotic use are now available from most European Union countries (see European Surveillance of Antibiotic Consumption, http://www.esac.ua.ac.be/main.aspx?c=* ESAC2&n=21600). From this and other investigations it was observed that antibiotic sales could vary more than fourfold between European countries. The figures in DDD per 1000 inhabitants per day were high for France (36.5), Spain (32.4), Portugal (28.8), and Belgium (26.7), and lower for the Netherlands (8.9), Denmark (11.3), Sweden (13.5), and Germany (13.6).

All these data on antibiotics consumption speak for stricter control of antibiotics use. This ought to limit overconsumption and diminish the total selection pressure toward resistance development. This is the most obvious and immediate way of at least slowing down the increase in antibiotics resistance among pathogenic bacteria. There are also two strong economic arguments for this. One is the high and increasing costs of antibiotics in the health care budget. The other is more difficult to discern. It is connected to higher care costs when antibiotic therapy fails because of resistance, higher infection control costs, and the necessity of using more expensive antibiotics. There are calculations of these costs by health care economists, who report them to be very high. There is a simple and mundane example of this. Treatment with linezolid (600 mg × 2) of an infection with methicillin-resistant staphylococci (MRSA) costs 83 times more than the corresponding treatment of methicillin-susceptible staphylococci with flucloxacillin (500 mg × 3). A slower selection of resistant bacteria would lead to substantial cost savings.

The speed of resistance development depends on the selection pressure of the distributed antibiotics; that is, the ubiquitous and increasing presence of antibiotics in the biosphere makes resistance a survival condition for an increasing number of bacteria, including commensal organisms, which are not pathogenic but will form a reservoir of resistance genes. It is then important to curb the use of antibiotics by using them only for the urgent treatment of pathogens causing infections. As a specific example, in the Stockholm (Sweden) area, amoxicillin and trimethoprim can no longer be used for empirical therapy for urinary tract infections with *Escherichia coli* before the resistance determinations are in from the bacteriological laboratory, because of widespread resistance. This bacterium is the pathogen found most commonly in these infections and is now very frequently resistant to the drugs mentioned. This is a great loss since amoxicillin and trimethoprim are inexpensive and efficient medicines and easy to handle.

CONTROL OF ANTIBIOTICS OVERUSE

The Council of Ministers of the European Union (EU) has issued several recommendations to the EU member states with the purpose of diminishing the use of antibiotics. Earlier, a large part of the antibiotics consumption was used as feed additives in husbandry and to some extent also in plant agriculture. The use in animals was based on the empirical but not completely understood observations that meat animals gained weight faster when given antibiotics in their fodder. It soon became clear, however, that this practice led to the spread of antibiotic resistance through the food chain into the general population. An example of this was the use of avoparcin, a glucopeptide, an analog to vancomycin (see Chapter 5). It was approved for growth promotion within the EU, particularly in the breeding of poultry. Substantial amounts were used. In one EU country in 1993, for example, 22 kg of vancomycin was employed in human therapy, while animal use consumed 19,000 kg of avoparcin. It soon became clear that this practice led to a widespread dissemination of vancomycin-resistant enterococci into the general population through the food chain. This was all the more frightening since vancomycin was looked upon as a drug of last resort in many cases of infectious disease. It is the drug of choice for the treatment of infections by methicillin-resistant staphylococci. Avoparcin was banned from livestock feed in the EU in 1997 after more than two decades of use. In monitoring the effect of the ban, a dramatic drop in the occurrence of vancomycin-resistant enterococci was seen in chickens and supermarket chicken meat. This could also be seen in stool samples from patients in which the prevalence of a key vancomycin resistance gene dropped from 5.7% to 0.8%, clearly demonstrating the good effect on resistance of restrictions in antibiotics distribution.

There is another interesting example of the consequences of using antibiotics for growth promotion in animal husbandry. It regards streptothricin, found in the *Streptomyces* screening efforts performed in Selman Waksman's laboratory described in Chapter 1. Streptothricin was found to be too toxic for human use but was used under the name nourseothricin for growth promotion in pig farms in the earlier East Germany. Soon after the introduction of streptothricin use, plasmid-borne resistance to streptothricin was observed in *E. coli* bacteria from nourseothricin-fed pigs and from employees and their family members on pig farms. Streptothricin resistance plasmids were furthermore found in *E. coli* isolated from the gut and from the urinary tracts of people with no connection to pig farms but living in villages and towns in an area where streptothricin was used in animal husbandry. These examples illustrate the rapid emergence of antimicrobial resistance and their powerful mechanisms of spread. Further investigation showed that the plasmid-borne gene mediating streptothricin resistance was in turn borne on a transposon on the plasmid. This transposon was also found to carry a gene for spectinomycin resistance (see Chapter 6). This means that the use of streptothricin not only selected for streptothricin resistance but also co-selected for resistance to an important antibacterial drug used in human medicine.

Antibiotics have also been distributed in plant agriculture: for example, in combatting the devastating plant disease of fire blight caused by the bacterium *Erwinia amylovora* and causing severe losses in apple and pear production. In the United States, 12 to 13 metric tons of streptomycin were used in the middle of the 1990s for the purpose of fighting this plant disease. Streptomycin resistance of a type recognized from human pathogens quickly appeared in *Erwinia amylovora*, and the practice was abandoned.

In later years, laws have been introduced in the EU to stop the use of antibiotics for growth promotion. This is a good example of cooperation within the EU to try to solve the ecological problem that the overuse of antibiotics really is. There also seems to be a remarkable overuse of antibiotics in health care. In this area, however, international laws for the strict use of antibiotics are difficult to introduce, since health care is a national responsibility within the EU. The national government within each member country is finally responsible for the health problem of increasing antibiotics resistance and the necessary restrictions in the distribution of antibiotics. Surveillance of resistance has to be improved and information campaigns initiated. There is an international organization for this purpose, the Alliance for the Prudent Use of Antibiotics (APUA, 75 Kneeland Street, Boston, MA 02111; web site: www.APUA.org; email: APUA@tufts.edu). This is an association with representatives from more than 20 different countries. It is dedicated to "preserving the power of antibiotics."

The total consumption of antibiotics is not alone to blame for the rapid development of resistance. This can be concluded from the resistance situation in developing countries such as Bangladesh, Nigeria, Sri Lanka, and Vietnam, where the consumption of antibiotics per inhabitant is less than a tenth of that in the industrialized world. Still, as described from sporadic reports, the resistance situation is much worse. This is due to the fact that antibiotic therapy cannot be well aimed because of insufficient resources for bacterial diagnosis and resistance determinations. Furthermore, antibiotics can be bought freely in the local market and are therefore often used incorrectly against insusceptible pathogens and in inadequate doses.

CHAPTER 3

SULFONAMIDES AND TRIMETHOPRIM

Sulfonamides and trimethoprim are at the extremes in the history of antibacterial agents for systemic use. As mentioned in Chapter 1, sulfonamide was the first selectively acting agent that could be used systemically. With the exception of linezolid, trimethoprim is in the truest sense the latest. Sulfonamide was introduced in 1935, and trimethoprim, around 1970. Of course, many different antibiotics have been launched and marketed during the long period since 1970, but all of them have been related to already existing antibiotics and have then become members of one or the other of the main antibiotic families (Chapter 11). Very importantly, cross resistance occurs within these families. The medical reasons for marketing these new family members have been that they have shown different spectra of activity: that is, higher efficiency toward specific pathogenic bacteria, and also, among these those that showed resistance against other members of the particular antibiotic family. However, in the latter case there are examples which show that the resistance

Antibiotics and Antibiotics Resistance, First Edition. Ola Sköld.
© 2011 John Wiley & Sons, Inc. Published 2011 by John Wiley & Sons, Inc.

within the family has adapted rapidly to the new agent (there are examples of this in Chapter 4).

The simple and inexpensive sulfonamides have been widely used and appreciated for many years. Resistance against them among pathogenic bacteria is now very common, however, and this development can be used as a clear and instructive example of the devaluation of the health care value of antibacterial agents by resistance. Next, we describe in detail mechanisms of sulfonamide resistance to illustrate the complexity of the resistance evolution at the molecular level. This description should also demonstrate the experimental approaches that can be used to elucidate mechanisms of resistance.

GENERAL ASPECTS REGARDING THE DEVELOPMENT OF RESISTANCE

To witness resistance development among bacteria is like looking at a gigantic laboratory of genetics. The very large distribution of antibiotics has meant a toxic shock, a dramatic environmental change for the microbial world. Bacteria have reacted by adaptation in the usual way: by evolution. We can look at it as Darwinian evolution in front of our eyes, which is accelerating, with further genetic mechanisms being selected for the horizontal spread of resistance genes. The bacterial world, including the pathogens, has developed molecular mechanisms for inactivating our antibacterial agents or evading their effect. The development of resistance among pathogenic bacteria has generally been astonishingly fast, which could be explained by the rapid growth of bacteria, allowing them to undergo evolution in a short time. This resistance evolution is not constant, but some resistance events have taken a long time to occur. It has no direction, but is opportunistic.

Furthermore, bacteria can manipulate their own genome, for example, by incorporating horizontally transferred genetic material carrying resistance genes, thereby increasing the speed of resistance development. This is an innate form of genetic engineering in which bacteria are able to adapt and use genetic mechanisms that have evolved earlier for general environmental adaptation, for the new purpose of spreading resistance genes between bacteria. This development has meant that many infectious diseases which earlier were easily handled with antibiotics are now more difficult to treat. The great triumph of medicine fades and we are forced to realize that the health standard that we have become used to regarding infectious diseases is not stable. The very large original value of antibiotics is gradually devalued. This process proceeds continuously and the general pattern is that resistance generally occurs between one or two years after the clinical introduction of a new antibiotic. This experience naturally curbs the interest of the pharmaceutical industry in pursuing research in this area. From an anthropomorphic perspective, however, no microbiologist can keep from admiring the ingenuity and efficiency that bacteria show in protecting themselves from the toxic effects of our antibiotics. How does this resistance evolution work, and what are the precise molecular mechanisms for antibiotics resistance?

New antibiotics in the true sense—that is, antibacterial agents with new points of attack at the molecular level—have been very limited in number in later years, and this is probably due to the tepid interest of the pharmaceutical industry in this area, for understandable reasons. The antibacterial treatment ought to be of short duration. If the antibacterial agent is effective, the infection heals quickly, and treatment can be terminated. Sales would be relatively small. There is no antibiotic among the 20 best-selling pharmaceuticals in Scandinavia. As mentioned earlier, resistance as a rule occurs within one or two years after the introduction of a new antibacterial agent. These circumstances mean that antibiotics are not very interesting from a marketing point of view.

SULFONAMIDES

The selective effect of sulfonamides on bacteria is due to their inhibiting effect on the formation of folic acid (Fig. 3.1), an important coenzyme of all living cells. Mammalian cells, our cells, are not endowed with that sequence of enzymic reactions necessary to synthesize folic acid, but rely on folic acid as a vitamin in our nourishment. Specifically, sulfonamides (formula **3-1**) were shown to interfere with the bacterial formation of folic acid by its structural similarity to the intermediate *p*-aminobenzoic acid (**3-2**). Sulfonamide is generally mentioned in the plural form because dozens of derivatives (modifications at the amino group at the sulfon residue) of Domag's original sulfanilamide have been synthesized through the years. All of these, however, are identical regarding their antibacterial effect. They have been synthesized only for pharmacokinetic reasons.

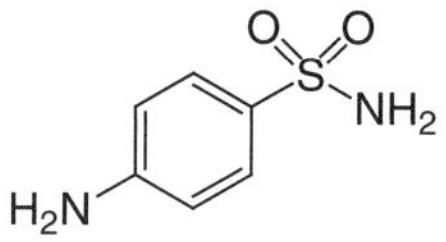

Sulfanilamide

3-1

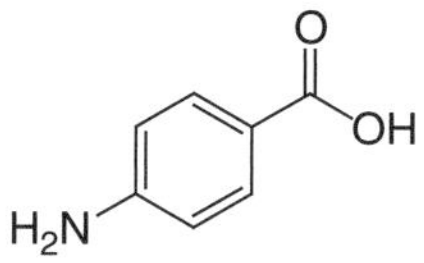

p-aminobenzoic acid

3-2

Sulfonamides as Remedies

Sulfonamides were widely used all over the world as cheap and effective remedies against bacterial infections. Today, however, the use of sulfonamides is very limited. In Scandinavia, the distribution of sulfonamides as a single drug for systemic use is presently nil. Aside from preparations for external use, as in ointments, the minimal distribution of sulfonamides that still occurs is in combination with trimethoprim.

There are three primary reasons for the almost nonexistent use of sulfonamides. First, other and in many cases more efficient antibacterial drugs became available through the decades following the introduction of sulfonamides in 1935. Second, resistance emerged rapidly in many pathogens. The third and most important reason, however, was the development of allergic side effects from the blood-forming organs and the skin in many patients. Systematic clinical studies have shown the occurrence of sulfonamide-induced blood dyscrasias, including aplastic anemia, at a frequency of 5.3 cases per million of defined daily doses and with a mortality of 17% in the affected group. As an example, in Sweden there was a trial between a patient association and a pharmaceutical company, culminating in a settlement with high compensation costs for damages, that more or less ended the systemic use of sulfonamides in that country. It could be debated whether the present situation, with its increasing frequencies of resistance against antibiotics, might not warrant a reintroduction of sulfonamides for use against that large number of pathogens that still are susceptible to sulfonamides, now with new knowledge and vigilance regarding allergic side effects.

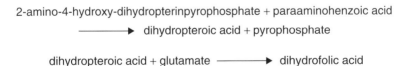

2-amino-4-hydroxy-dihydropterinpyrophosphate + paraaminobenzoic acid
⟶ dihydropteroic acid + pyrophosphate

dihydropteroic acid + glutamate ⟶ dihydrofolic acid

FIGURE 3.1 Point of action of sulfonamides on the folic acid synthesis of bacteria, the last two steps of which are shown schematically. The next-to-last step is catalyzed by the enzyme dihydropteroate synthase, which is the target of sulfonamides.

Resistance to Sulfonamide

As mentioned, an early reason for the diminished use of sulfon-amides was the rapid development of resistance in many pathogens: for example, streptococci, meningococci, and gonococci. Resistance toward sulfonamides is now also very common among gram-negative enterobacteria infecting the urinary tract. The molecular mechanisms of sulfonamide resistance differ markedly between different bacteria and have become investigated only in relatively recent years. The simplest mechanism includes mutational changes in the sulfonamide target enzyme dihydropteroate synthase (Fig. 3.1) that limit binding of the drug and thus mitigate the competition with the normal substrate p-aminobenzoic acid. Dihydropteroate synthase catalyzes the next-to-last step in the enzymic pathway leading to folic acid. In this step the pteridin nucleus of folic acid is linked to p-aminobenzoic acid. The structural similarity between sulfonamide and p-aminobenzoic acid and the high affinity of sulfonamide to the enzyme effects a competitive inhibition of dihydropteroate formation and, in turn, of folic acid formation. If a spontaneous mutation hits the chromosomal gene expressing dihydropteroate synthase, changing the enzyme structure such that it binds sulfonamide less tightly, the compe-tition with p-aminobenzoic acid will be less pronounced, and its host then shows sulfonamide resistance. This phenomenon was shown in a simple laboratory experiment where *E. coli* bacteria were spread on agar plates containing inhibiting concentrations of sulfonamide. Single colonies, about one in 100 million of totally spread bacteria, showed resistance and grew out to colonies. The nucleotide sequence of the dihydropteroate synthase gene in those resistant bacteria showed that a spontaneous point mutation had occurred, exchanging one nucleotide and in turn exchanging one amino acid in the enzyme expressed.

Closer studies of this resistance enzyme showed a 150-fold increase in the value of the inhibition constant (K_i). This means that the concentration of sulfonamide has to be increased 150-fold compared to that needed for the same inhibition of the nonmutated enzyme. It could be seen, however, that the host bacterium had had to pay a price for its resistance, in that the mutationally changed enzyme needed a 10-fold higher concentration of its normal substrate, p-aminobenzoic acid, to function optimally (a 10-fold increase in the K_m). The mutated enzyme also showed temperature sensitivity. The presence of sulfonamide creates an acute survival situation in which a mutationally changed enzyme is selected to help bacteria survive, but at the price of a less efficient enzyme differing from the optimal structure selected during the long evolution of bacteria. This would mean that bacteria reverting to their original susceptibility ought to be selected in the absence of sulfonamide. These arguments regarding molecular evolution and antibiotics resistance are very important for the medical assessment of resistance against antibacterial agents in health care (see Chapter 11): for example, the question of whether antibiotic resistance seen in clinical contexts incurs a fitness cost on the host bacterium, thus counterselecting against resistant bacteria in the absence of antibiotics.

Resistance to Sulfonamides in *Neisseria meningitidis*

We now provide a detailed characterization of sulfonamide resistance in *Neisseria meningitidis*. It includes kinetic characteristics of those resistance variations of dihydropteroate synthase observed in clinical isolates of resistant pathogens, studied with site-directed mutagenesis. It is meant as an illustration at the molecular level of what has happened to a cheap and efficient antibacterial agent under the evolution of resistance.

After sulfonamides were introduced for clinical use in the 1930s, they were frequently used in both prophylaxis and treatment of infectious meningitis, a disease which without treatment shows a very high mortality. The etiological agent, *N. meningitidis*, soon developed sulfonamide resistance. This and the emergence of other more efficient agents has meant that sulfonamides have not been used for this disease for decades, which ought to mean that sulfonamide-resistant isolates of *N. meningitidis* should not exist today according to the argument described earlier for mutational sulfonamide resistance. They do, however, and are in fact common among present-day isolates of this pathogen. This means that they have not been selected away in the absence of sulfonamides. This in turn means that sulfonamide resistance has not hindered the resistant strains in their growth competition with their susceptible relatives. The fitness cost of resistance assumed must have been compensated in some way. The resistance remaining today can be looked at as a scar left by an earlier antibacterial treatment frequently used. It is an illustration of how our use of antibacterial agents changes bacterial evolution.

A closer study of the sulfonamide resistance mechanism among meningococci revealed surprisingly large differences between resistant and susceptible isolates in the gene expressing dihydropteroate synthase, the target enzyme of sulfonamides. Nucleotide sequence determinations of the *fol*P gene, as it is called, from many susceptible and resistant isolates showed that there are two classes of resistance genes. In one of these the resistance *fol*P gene differed by 10% in its sequence from that of susceptible isolates. This very large difference cannot be due to mutations accrued over time but must reflect a horizontal transfer of *fol*P DNA between bacteria. This could be understood as spontaneous transformation, since *Neisseria* bacteria have the ability to take up DNA from relatives and incorporate it in their genomes. This ability gives *Neisseria* bacteria access to a common stock of genes that is much larger than that of the single species.

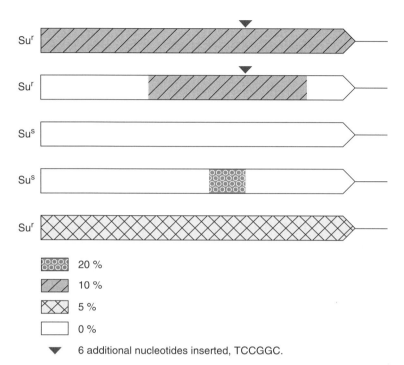

FIGURE 3.2 Sulfonamide resistance in *N. meningitidis*. Comparisons of the nucleotide sequences of *fol*P genes from different sulfonamide-resistant and sulfonamide-susceptible clinical isolates of *N. meningitidis*. The sequence differences in the stylized gene representations are denoted by differently marked areas and percentages. *Su*^{r}, the resistance gene; *Su*^{s}, the susceptibility gene. The six extra nucleotides mentioned in the text are located at the triangle symbol.

Among the sulfonamide-resistant strains there were also *fol*P genes showing a mosaic of sorts, where only the central part corresponded to the resistance gene, while the outer parts were identical to those of a susceptible *fol*P (Fig. 3.2).

Other *Neisseria* species are most likely to be the origin of the resistance gene. In these species, sulfonamide-resistant dihydropteroate synthases could be occurring naturally; that is, they could have evolved structurally as not being able to bind sulfonamides. There is a parallel to this in plasmid-borne genes for sulfonamide resistance, described later in the chapter. As an alternative, the sulfonamide resistance could have developed in harmless commensals and later, transferred into pathogenic *Neisseria* bacteria (this is developed a little bit more later). The idea of horizontal transfer of resistance-mediating DNA is supported by the observation of an 80-base pair DNA fragment from the corresponding part of *fol*P in *N. gonorrhoeae* showing a 20% sequence difference from *N. meningitidis* and located in a sulfonamide-susceptible strain of *N. meningitidis*. This is an illustration of the horizontal mobility of genetic material between related *Neisseria* species. This mosaic formation in *Neisseria* is shown in Figure 3.3.

It could be added, speculatively, that the horizontal mobility described must be regulated in some way lest the species identity be jeopardized. On the other hand, it could be suggested that the selection pressure of our antibiotics is so strong that it could force itself through this regulation and, in the long run, influence the species barriers between pathogenic bacteria. The sulfonamide resistance gene in *N. meningitidis* described earlier has one additional characteristic. It has six extra nucleotides inserted at one point in its sequence, corresponding to two extra amino acids, glycine and serine, in the dihydropteroate synthase expressed (Fig. 3.2). If these two amino acids are removed experimentally by site-directed mutagenesis, the dihydropteroate synthase expressed becomes sulfonamide susceptible, implying that they are decisive for resistance. In the experimental system for this determination the *fol*P gene has been moved from the *Neisseria* chromosome to a small plasmid, which in turn was introduced in an experimental bacterium. In a test tube system such as that, the *fol*P DNA can be taken out, manipulated by site-directed mutagenesis, and inserted in an experimental bacterium whose sulfonamide susceptibility can then be determined.

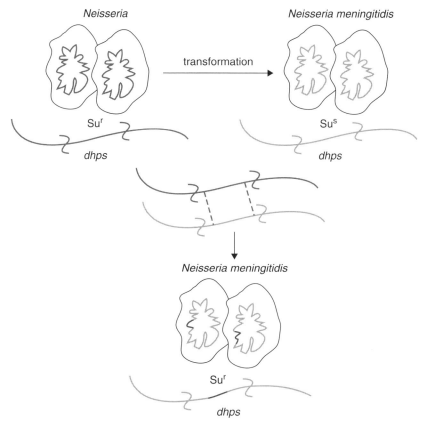

FIGURE 3.3 Transformation of sulfonamide resistance into *N. meningitidis*. Schematic illustration of the horizontal transfer of genetic material between *Neisseria* species, which after recombination gives rise to sulfonamide resistance (cf. Fig. 3.2); *dhps*, dihydropteroate synthase; *Su*^{r}, sulfonamide resistant; *Su*^{s}, sulfonamide susceptible.

The other class of sulfonamide-resistant *N. meningitidis* show a 5% difference in their *folP* nucleotide sequence compared to that of a susceptible strain, and also lack the two extra amino acids, serine and glycine, in their expressed dihydropteroate synthase. Several of these resistance genes are identical between different resistant bacterial isolates but different from that of a susceptible isolate. This again implies a horizontal spread of resistance, in this case of the entire target enzyme gene (Fig. 3.2).

Characterization of the Sulfonamide-Resistant Dihydropteroate Synthase in N. meningitidis

Next we look in detail at the differences in amino acid sequence between dihydropteroate synthase from sulfonamide-susceptible meningococci and the corresponding resistant meningococci. We describe the mechanism as completely as possible and as a general example of resistance evolution in bacteria. A comparison of the amino acid sequences between susceptible and resistant enzymes, respectively, showed about 20 specific differences. Three of these affected amino acids, which have been identified in the same position in all known bacterial dihydropteroate synthases, indicating their role in the basic function of the enzyme (Fig. 3.4). One of those was Phe31 (phenylalanine; 31 is the consecutive number from the amino end of the peptide), which in the resistance enzyme is substituted for by Leu (leucine).

This is functionally the same amino acid exchange that was involved in the spontaneous mutation to sulfonamide resistance in *E. coli*, described earlier in the chapter, where the corresponding phenylalanine has the consecutive number 28, which then gives Phe28Leu (phenylalanine in position 28 exchanged for leucine). In addition to Leu31, the resistance enzyme in meningococci also has Ser84 and Cys194 as exchanged amino acids. By site-directed mutagenesis experiments in vitro, these amino acid exchanges were systematically restored to the amino acid pattern of the susceptible enzyme. When Leu31 for resistance was changed to Phe31 of the susceptible enzyme, the resistance decreased 25-fold; that is, the (minimum inhibitory concentration (MIC) value) for sulfonamide decreased from 0.5 mM to less than 0.02 mM. When, correspondingly, the Cys194 of resistance

				K_m	K_i	MIC
				µM	µM	µM
Su^s	Phe	Pro	Gly	0.5	0.4	< 0.02
	31	84	194			
Su^r	Leu	Ser	Cys	2.9	218	> 0.5
	Phe	Ser	Cys	0.5	0.6	< 0.02
	Leu	Ser	Gly	0.6	5	0.12
	Leu	Pro	Cys	6.9	626	> 0.5

FIGURE 3.4 Sulfonamide resistance in *N. meningitidis*. The effect of specific amino acid changes on meningococcal resistance to sulfonamide. A stylized representation of the dihydropteroate synthase with the three amino acids that are important for resistance, marked by their sequence numbers. Above the protein symbol the amino acid configuration for susceptibility, *Su^s* is given, and below the protein symbol there is the configuration for resistance, *Su^r*. To the right there are the values determined for the Michaelis constant (K_m), the inhibition constant (K_i), and the MIC value for sulfonamide, in this case sulfathiazole. The different amino acid configurations show the effect of systematic amino acid exchanges by site-directed mutagenesis. See the text for further details.

was exchanged for the Gly194 of susceptibility, the MIC value for sulfonamide decreased from 0.5 mM to 0.12 mM. Both of these amino acid changes are thus closely related to resistance. It could be added that both Leu31 and Cys194 are located in highly conserved areas of the enzyme peptide; that is, they are very similar, if not identical, among all known bacterial dihydropteroate synthases, which in turn ought to mean that they are involved in the catalytic function of the enzyme. Finally, when Ser84 for resistance was changed to Pro84 corresponding to susceptibility, no effect on MIC could be observed.

Quantitative measurements of enzyme kinetics were performed to further characterize sulfonamide resistance. In these experiments, the artificially mutated meningococcal gene for dihydropteroate synthase, borne on a small plasmid, was allowed to express itself in a laboratory strain of E. *coli* in which the chromosomal gene for dihydropteroate synthase had been inactivated by a partial deletion. Extracts from such a system would thus contain only meningococcal enzyme, and sulfonamide effects on mutated forms of this enzyme could then be measured specifically and precisely. It was shown that the K_i value for sulfonamide (in this case, sulfathiazol), which is a quantitative measure of the affinity of the inhibitor for the enzyme, showed good correlation with the MIC values assessed (Fig. 3.4). The amino acid exchange of resistance Leu31 to susceptibility 31Phe caused an almost 400-fold decrease in the K_i value for sulfonamide. At the same time, a sixfold decrease in the K_m value for the normal substrate of p-aminobenzoic acid could be observed. Also, changing the Cys194 of resistance to Gly194 of susceptibility resulted in a substantial decrease in K_i, whereas changing resistance Ser84 to susceptibility 84Pro increased the K_i value for sulfonamide threefold and also increased the K_m value for p-aminobenzoic acid twofold. The resistance Ser84 can be regarded as a compensatory amino acid exchange, stabilizing the resistance enzyme to show the same efficiency as that of the original sensitive enzyme.

Characterization of the Other Sulfonamide-Resistant Dihydropteroate Synthase in N. meningitidis

That other type of sulfonamide resistance enzyme with the two extra amino acids inserted in its peptide sequence described earlier in the chapter was subjected to a detailed characterization regarding kinetics and structure. When the six extra nucleotides corresponding to the inserted amino acids Ser195 and Gly196 were removed by site-directed mutagenesis, the K_i value for sulfonamide decreased 10-fold, resulting in susceptibility. At the same time, however, there was a 10-fold increase in the K_m value for the normal substrate p-aminobenzoic acid. This must mean that the two extra amino acids alone do not mediate resistance but that there are also other and compensatory amino acid changes, which all together result in a resistant enzyme with the same efficiency as that of the original susceptibility enzyme. This is illustrated further by an experiment in which the two extra amino acids Ser195 and Gly196 were inserted artificially in a susceptibility enzyme. This did not result in resistance, however, but affected the K_m value for the normal substrate with a 100-fold increase; that is, it resulted in an enzyme so inefficient that it cannot support a living bacterium. The resistance enzyme structure thus seems to be more complicated than can be explained by the experiments and observations described, which, however, seem to imply that resistance was the property of other bacterial species, later moved to pathogenic meningococci by transformation and recombination. This is supported further by the isolation of sulfonamide-resistant *Neisseria* commensals (i.e., nonpathogenic *Neisseria* bacteria) described from throat samples of outpatients. Since, as mentioned earlier, sulfonamides are no longer used for systemic treatment, it can be concluded that those throat samples were isolated from patients not lately exposed to sulfonamides. The isolated commensals often showed high resistance to sulfonamides and were identified as *N. subflava, N. sicca,* and *N. mucosa*. Their *folP* genes showed resistance characteristics that were very similar to those described for the resistant pathogenic *N. meningitidis*. They could be suspected to be the origin of resistance in pathogenic meningococci, but experiments to transfer resistance from commensals to pathogens by tranformation have not been successful. This is probably because the regulatory mechanisms for spontaneous transformation retain the specificity of species. However, it could be speculated that the earlier ubiqitous use of sulfonamides could have created such a strong selection pressure that those regulatory mechanisms were overcome by sheer selection force.

This rather detailed description of sulfonamide resistance among meningococci might serve as an illustration of the complexity of resistance mechanisms and their spread among pathogenic bacteria. Also, it could illustrate that in most cases, resistance is not a fitness cost in the life and growth of bacteria, which in turn means that resistance is in most cases probably not spontaneously reversible. The sulfonamide example could raise interesting speculations regarding antibiotics resistance in general. The resistance *fol*P described could have evolved by an evolutionary process under the large selection pressure of the ubiquitous use of sulfonamides since the middle of the 1930s. Alternatively, it could represent an evolutionary dihydropteroate synthase structure that by chance has a very low affinity for the *p*-aminobenzoic acid analog sulfonamide. Also speculatively, there is a possibility that there are sulfonamide analogs (salicylates?) in nature against which bacteria have developed protection mechanisms, which in turn have been forced into pathogens by the human-made selection pressure of sulfonamides.

Resistance to Sulfonamides in *Streptococcus pyogenes*

The vicious pathogen *S. pyogenes*, which in earlier times often led to life-threatening septicemias among patients, was one of the first pathogens treated successfully with sulfonamides, 80 years ago. Sulfonamides were also used for prophylaxis against streptococcal infections among soldiers in military training camps during World War II. Failures of this prophylaxis due to the appearance of resistant streptococcal strains were reported as early as 1946. Streptococcal treatment with sulfonamides then stopped, partly because of resistance, but mainly because of the introduction of penicillin, which very soon turned out to be superior for streptococcal treatment, and the mechanism of the early sulfonamide resistance was not investigated and described until later years. It ought to be mentioned that penicillin is still the best agent for the treatment of streptococcal infections. As a lucky exception from the empirical rule of rapid development of resistance, *S. pyogenes* has kept its susceptibility to penicillin, which can still be used to treat infections that it has caused. The reason for this fortunate condition is unknown.

Despite the fact that sulfonamides have not long been used for the treatment of streptococcal infections, sulfonamide resistance is common among present isolates of *S. pyogenes*. This is a further interesting illustration of the nonreversibility of resistance in the absence of the selecting effect of the drug. The drug-resistant phenotypes do not seem to be at any disadvantage in competition with their drug-susceptible relatives. Sulfonamide-resistant strains of *S. pyogenes* were shown to have very high resistance, some of them with MIC values of 1 mg/mL. The mechanism of resistance in *S. pyogenes* turned out to be related to the sulfonamide resistance of *N. meningitidis*, in that it is based on the horizontal transfer of genetic material. Detailed studies have shown that the *fol*P in susceptible and highly resistant isolates differed by 13.8% in nucleotide sequence. This difference is too large to be due to accumulated mutations. The resistance gene must have been introduced by transformation or transduction. The sequence analysis of the complete genome shows that *S. pyogenes* contains an inducible prophage, indicating the possibility of phage-mediated transduction. Further studies on sulfonamide resistance in *S. pyogenes*, including nucleotide sequence determination of the genes neighboring the sulfonamide target gene *fol*P in the folate operon, demonstrated an overall difference of 15% in the nucleotide sequence. More specifically, areas of different nucleotide sequences were scattered over the folate operon in a mosaic fashion, indicating horizontal transfer of foreign DNA of unknown origin. The *folP* gene of resistant isolates showed different areas of foreign DNA in different isolates. These areas could be identical within groups of resistant isolates. The import of foreign resistance-mediating DNA into the sulfonamide target gene *folP* is thus an analogy to the sulfonamide resistance described in meningococci.

Resistance to Sulfonamides in *Campylobacter jejuni*

Sulfonamide resistance is commonly found in clinical isolates of *C. jejuni*. It is mediated by chromosomal point mutations, but in a rather complicated pattern. The sulfonamide target gene *folP* was found to be very large compared to that of other bacteria and also quite similar to the corresponding gene of the peptic ulcer bacterium, *Helicobacter pylori*. The *folP* from a resistant isolate of *C. jejuni* differed by four mutations from that of a corresponding susceptible isolate. The ensuing amino acid changes in the sulfonamide target enzyme, dihydropteroate synthase, mediated a distinct effect on the sulfonamide sensitivity of the enzyme. The K_i value for sulfonamide increased from $0.5\,\mu M$ with the susceptibility enzyme to $500\,\mu M$ for the resistance enzyme.

Resistance to Sulfonamides in *Streptococcus pneumoniae*

In this pathogen, sulfonamide resistance is mediated by a different type of chromosomal change. Originally, a spontaneous laboratory mutant of this bacterium was found to contain a six-nucleotide repeat in the sulfonamide target gene, *folP*, which in turn mediated an amino acid repeat of isoleucine and glutamic acid in the dihydropteroate synthase expressed from the gene. This could significantly alter the tertiary structure of the enzyme protein, which was later borne out by crystallographic studies. Clinical isolates of sulfonamide-resistant *S. pneumoniae* showed amino acid duplications at several different locations in the protein, which indicates several independent changes to resistance. Finally, the ileu–glu repeat studied originally was also observed in a clinical isolate of *S. pneumoniae*, and when this repeat was removed by site-directed mutagenesis, susceptibility ensued. Transformation experiments demonstrated that the duplication was sufficient to confer the sulfonamide resistance observed. Enzyme kinetic studies on the dihydropteroate synthase after removal of the repeat by site-directed mutagenesis, showed the K_i for sulfonamide to drop from 18 μM to 0.4 μM (i.e., 35-fold) while the K_m for *p*-aminobenzoic acid decreased 2.5-fold. The enzyme characteristics for the artificially mutated strain were identical to those of susceptible strains, demonstrating that the duplication is sufficient for resistance. The fitness cost of resistance seems to be low, as reflected in the small increase in the K_m value. The small but discernible increase indicates the absence of compensatory mutations. Still it could be enough for counterselecting resistant strains in the absence of the drug and might lead to an argument regarding the much-debated problem of drug resistance reversibility.

Resistance to Sulfonamides in *Pneumocystis jiroveci (carinii)*

This pathogenic organism is a fungus causing life-threatening pneumonia in immunosuppressed patients. Co-trimoxazole, the combination of sulfonamide (sulfamethoxazole) and trimethoprim, has been the drug of choice for the prophylaxis and treatment of this disease. Lifelong prophylaxis was often recommended for HIV-positive patients. The antipneumocystis effect of this drug combination is due primarily to the sulfonamide component, since studies on the trimethoprim target, dihydrofolate reductase, of this organism have shown trimethoprim to be a very poor inhibitor of this enzyme in it. Dapsone (4,4′-diaminodiphenyl sulfone; **3-3**) a sulfone drug acting microbiologically as a sulfonamide, has also frequently been used to treat this infection.

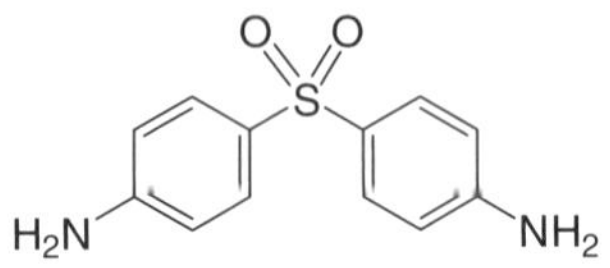

Dapsone

3-3

Pneumocystis jiroveci has thus been heavily exposed to sulfonamide, with an increasing prevalence of resistance mutations in its *folP* gene as a consequence. The human *P. jiroveci* cannot be cultured, and its dihydropteroate synthase protein is not readily available for study, but the corresponding *folP* sequence is known and two sulfonamide resistance mutations have been defined. They appear either as single or double mutations in the same isolate. There is thus the important question of whether the emergence of resistance mutations is the result of transmission between patients or arise and are selected within an individual patient under the pressure of sulfonamide or dapsone treatment. The latter interpretation has been favored (i.e., the mutants are selected within a given patient), and the mutations mentioned may be associated with reactivation of the infection.

Resistance to Sulfonamides in *Staphylococcus aureus* and *S. haemolyticus*

Chromosomal mutations in *folP* in an erratic pattern are involved. Nucleotide sequencing could discern four different mutational patterns and identify as many as 14 amino acid changes in the development of resistance. A simple interpretation of their role in resistance has not been possible.

Resistance to Sulfonamides in *Mycobacterium leprae*

Dapsone (4,4'-diaminodiphenyl sulfone), microbiologically a sulfonamide (see **3-3**), has been a standard remedy in leprosy treatment for a long time, and sulfonamide resistance in the form of three chromosomal mutations in the *fol*P gene has been defined. At present, rifampicin (see Chapter 9) is the drug of choice for the treatment of leprosy.

Plasmid-Borne Resistance to Sulfonamides

Sulfonamide insusceptibility was one of the first antibiotic resistance traits found to be transferable (see Chapter 10). Since sulfonamide is a synthetic antibacterial agent, resistance by plasmid-mediated drug-degrading or drug-modifying enzymes was not to be expected. Instead, nonallelic, drug-resistant varieties of the chromosomal dihydropteroate synthase drug target enzyme were found to mediate high levels of sulfonamide resistance (Fig. 3.5). Three types of plasmid-borne genes expressing such varieties are known: *sul*1, *sul*2, and *sul*3. These three genes differ among themselves (40% similarity at the amino acid level). Their origins are not known. The occurrence of these three plasmid-borne genes is the most common form of sulfonamide resistance among clinically isolated enterobacteria. Remarkably, only *sul*1 and *sul*2 or both were long found in isolates of sulfonamide-resistant enterobacteria from various parts of the world. This is in contrast to trimethoprim resistance, described later in the chapter, at which more than 20 different plasmid-borne resistance genes have been found and characterized. The reason for this could be limited possibilities of configuration variation in the catalytic center of dihydropteroate synthase. The sulfonamide-resistant enzyme must be able to distinguish between its normal substrate *p*-aminobenzoic acid and the structurally very similar sulfonamide (see **3-1** and **3-2**). The enzymes

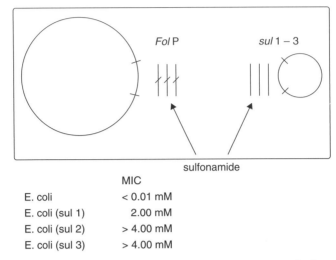

	MIC
E. coli	< 0.01 mM
E. coli (sul 1)	2.00 mM
E. coli (sul 2)	> 4.00 mM
E. coli (sul 3)	> 4.00 mM

FIGURE 3.5 Plasmid-borne resistance to sulfonamides. Stylized representation of a gram-negative bacterium. The *fol*P gene is marked on the large circular chromosome representing the chromosomal sulfonamide-sensitive dihydropteroate synthase. Plasmid-borne genes for sulfonamide resistance, *sul*, express dihydropteroate synthases that are insusceptible to inhibition by sulfonamides. Minimum inhibitory concentrations for sulfonamides are given for the different plasmid-mediated dihydropteroate synthases.

expressed from *sul*1 and *sul*2 bind the normal substrate well, showing low K_m values (0.6 µM), and can still resist very high concentrations of sulfonamide. In particular, *sul*2 shows a sharp acuity in its ability to distinguish between normal substrate and sulfonamide. It mediates resistance to very high concentrations of sulfonamide (>4.00 mM).

In a study from the early 1990s, a large number of sulfonamide-resistant clinical isolates of enterobacteria from different parts of the world were shown to harbor either *sul*1 or *sul*2 or both as plasmid-borne genes mediating sulfonamide resistance. The frequency of occurrence of *sul*1 and *sul*2 was about the same. The relatively recent finding of *sul*3, originally on plasmids in *E. coli* isolates from swine, but later also from human isolates, is very interesting in this context. In addition to being borne on plasmids, the three *sul* genes have further genetic mechanisms available for their rapid spread. Regarding *sul*1, for example, it is almost always located in an integron of the Tn21 type (Chapter 10) together with other resistance genes. The *sul*2 gene is usually found on small and movable plasmids of the *inc*Q type. The *sul*3 observed later is mediated by a composite transposon with flanks of known insertion sequences (Chapter 10).

As mentioned, the two resistance genes *sul*1 and *sul*2 occurred in about the same frequencies among clinical isolates of sulfonamide-resistant enterobacteria. In a later study from the United Kingdom regarding sulfonamide resistance in *E. coli*, it was shown that the frequency of sulfonamide resistance among these bacteria had increased despite the fact that sulfonamides have long not been used for systemic treatment in the UK. Furthermore, it was seen that the relative frequency of *sul*2 had increased and that it was now to be found mostly on large transferable plasmids (Chapter 10) together with many other resistance genes. The explanation of this unexpected phenomenon could be that *sul*2 had become associated with other resistance genes and then been selected via the use of other antibacterial agents. This is an important interpretation, since it bears on the spread of resistance by linkage between different resistance genes. Selection for one resistance could select for others as well. Another, location of *sul*2, found relatively recently, is on the chromosome of *Haemophilus influenzae*. This is a good illustration of the very high mobility of resistance genes.

TRIMETHOPRIM

Trimethoprim (**3-4**) is related to sulfonamides in the sense that it interferes with folate metabolism (Fig. 3.6). With its

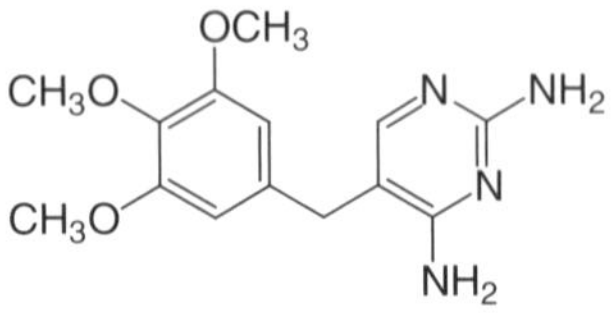

Trimethoprim

3-4

2,4-diaminopyrimidine structure, it is an analog of the folic acid pterin moiety and competitively inhibits the reduction of dihydrofolate (**3-5**) to tetrahydrofolate (**3-6**) by the enzyme dihydrofolate reductase. This is in analogy with the antifolate cytostatic drugs aminopterin (**3-7**) and methotrexate (**3-8**), the

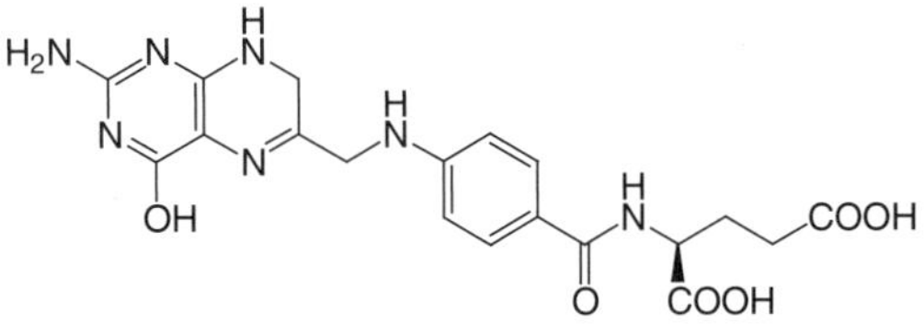

Dihydrofolic acid

3-5

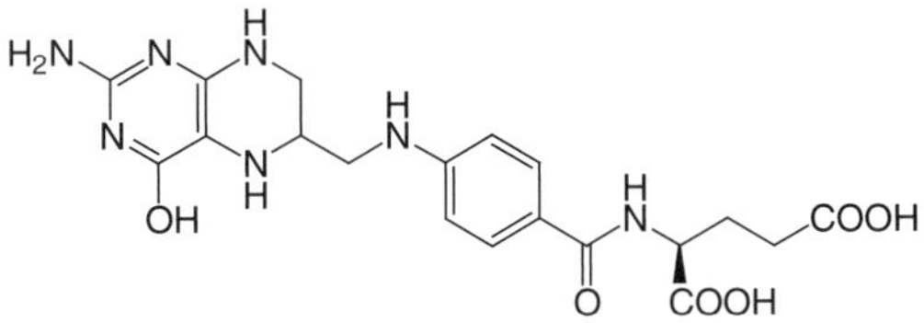

Tetrahydrofolic acid

3-6

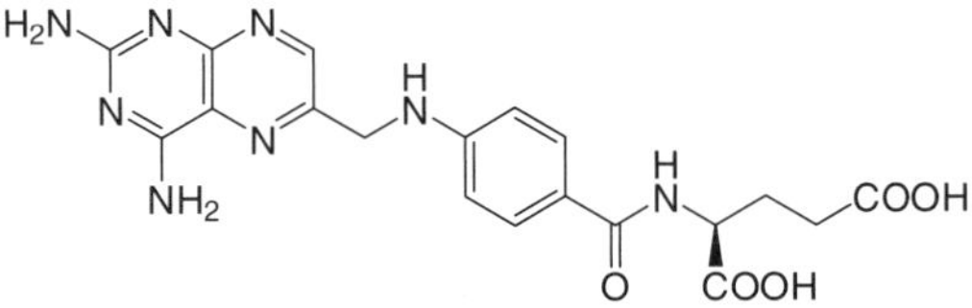

Aminopterin

3-7

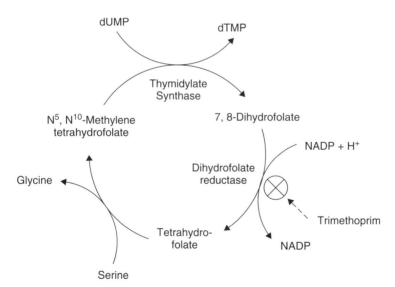

Methotrexate

3-8

latter having been used as a cytostatic agent since the 1950s. Methotrexate and aminopterin cannot be used as antibacterial agents, however, since they are not selective for bacteria. Inhibition of dihydrofolate reductase leads to a lack of tetrahydrofolate, which is an important coenzyme, for example, in the bacterial synthesis of DNA-thymine.

Trimethoprim was identified as a selectively acting antibacterial agent in large screening experiments, where great numbers

FIGURE 3.6 Role of tetrahydrofolate in the synthesis of DNA thymine. At the methylation reaction the tetrahydrofolate is oxidized and its rereduction by dihydrofolate reductase is inhibited by trimethoprim.

of folic acid analogs were tested systematically for the selective action on bacteria. The selective action of trimethoprim on bacterial dihydrofolate reductase, leaving mammalian enzymes untouched, allows the clinical use of trimethoprim as an antibacterial drug inhibiting bacterial dihydrofolate reductases at very low concentrations. As a matter of fact, trimethoprim does not interfere with human dihydrofolate reductase even at concentrations 10,000-fold higher than the usually very low MIC values found for most bacteria. There is a structural explanation for this, elucidated by x-ray crystallography studies, showing that trimethoprim fits well into the nucleotide binding site of the dihydrofolate reductase from, for example, *E. coli*, but not in the corresponding site of the mammalian enzyme. Trimethoprim has a broad antibacterial spectrum. This can vary slightly with analogs of trimethoprim such as iclaprim (**3-9**) and epiroprim (**3-10**). In this context, pyrimethamine could be mentioned. It is

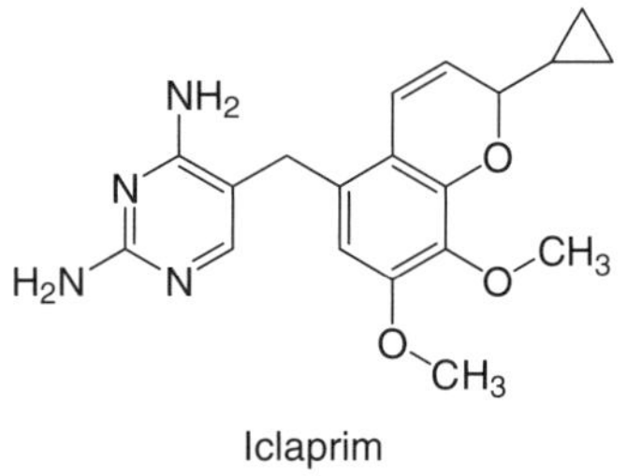

Iclaprim

3-9

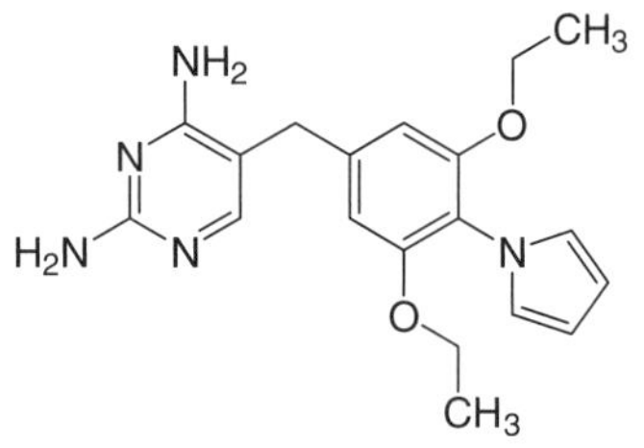

Epiroprim

3-10

structurally closely related to trimethoprim but is poorly active against bacterial dihydrofolate reductases and leaves the human enzyme unaffected, but has a strong inhibitory effect on the dihydrofolate reductase of the malaria plasmodium and has a good and specific effect in the treatment of malaria.

Since sulfonamides and trimethoprim attack successive steps in the same enzymic pathway leading to tetrahydrofolate, there is a synergistic effect that has been exploited in the combination drug co-trimoxazole, which contains trimethoprim in combination with the sulfonamide sulfamethoxazole. This sulfonamide was chosen for the combination in order to match the pharmacokinetic properties of trimethoprim. Trimethoprim was introduced around 1970 as a useful antibacterial agent for systemic use. It can be said that aside from linezolid from the 1990s (Chapter 7), trimethoprim was the last new antibacterial agent in the true sense of the word: new in the sense that its molecular mechanism of antibacterial action had not been used earlier. Trimethoprim has been much appreciated as an inexpensive and efficient agent in treating, for example, bacterial infections of the urinary tract, and has been used widely and extensively. Resistance is common, unfortunately, and is gaining in frequency.

Innate Resistance to Trimethoprim

Certain pathogens such as *C. jejuni* and *H. pylori* are naturally resistant to trimethoprim. Astonishing results from rather recent research have shown that these bacteria have no chromosomal gene (*fol*A) for dihydrofolate reductase and thus do not offer any target for antifolates. Tetrahydrofolate-borne one-carbon units are required for RNA, DNA, and protein synthesis. The dominant requirement for reduced folates in actively growing bacteria is for the methylation of deoxyuridylic acid to deoxythymidine-5'-monophosphate (thymidylate) under the catalysis of thymidylate synthase (*thy*A). In this process the methylene tetrahydrofolate gets oxidized to dihydrofolate, which is then reduced to tetrahydrofolate by dihydrofolate reductase expressed from *fol*A, which all *thy*A-carrying bacteria also contain (Fig. 3.6). There is, however, a rather recently discovered pathway for thymidylate synthesis, catalyzed by the protein product of *thy*X, which does not involve the oxidation of tetrahydrofolate but in which reduced flavin nucleotides ($FADH_2$) have an obligatory role. The *thy*X-carrying *C. jejuni* and *H. pylori* would then seem to be able to do without *fol*A, and thus without dihydrofolate reductase, the target of trimethoprim. They use alternative cofactors in the life-supporting synthesis of DNA-thymine. This means that tetrahydrofolate is not oxidized at the methylation reaction, leading to thymidylate in these bacteria. Dihydrofolate is not produced, which obviates the rereduction catalyzed by dihydrofolate reductase.

Chromosomal Resistance to Trimethoprim

Resistance to trimethoprim by mutations in the *fol*A gene expressing the trimethoprim target enzyme dihydrofolate reductase is known from several pathogenic bacteria. One example of this is a clinical isolate of *E. coli*, which overproduced its chromosomal didrofolate reductase several hundredfold by a combination of four types of mutations enhancing its expression. One was a promoter up mutation in the -35 region of the promoter; the second was an insertion of one base pair, increasing the distance between the -10 region of the promoter and the start codon. There were also several mutations optimizing the ribosome binding site, and finally, there were mutations in the structural gene, effecting changes to more frequently used codons. This increase in the intracellular enzyme level together with a mutational amino acid exchange substituting a Gly for a Try in the enzyme protein, thereby mediating a threefold increase in the K_i for the drug were thought to explain the high resistance (MIC$>$1000 μg/mL) observed for the isolate mentioned. The changes described represent a remarkable evolutionary adaptation to the antibacterial action of trimethoprim.

A similar type of chromosomal resistance to trimethoprim was observed in *H. influenzae*, where differences in the promoter region and in the structural gene for dihydrofolate reductase could be observed between trimethoprim susceptible and resistant isolates. Different parts of the structural gene were changed in different isolates and also in the C-terminal area, which is not known to participate in substrate or trimethoprim binding. These changes were suggested to involve alterations in the secondary structure, mediating a decrease in trimethoprim binding.

Chromosomal resistance to trimethoprim in *S. pneumoniae* is rather common. Resistant strains were shown to express dihydrofolate reductases, which resisted trimethoprim concentrations 50-fold higher than those inhibiting the corresponding enzyme from susceptible bacteria. In a study of 11 trimethoprim-resistant isolates, a substantial variability was seen in the nucleotide sequences of their dihydrofolate reductases genes. The resistant isolates could be divided into two groups with six amino acid changes in common. One of the two groups showed two extra changes, and the other, six additional changes. The high number of changes indicated a horizontal transfer of resistance genes. This interpretation is supported experimentally by the ability of chromosomal DNA from resistant isolates and cloned polymerase chain reaction products from resistance strains to transform a susceptible strain of *S. pneumoniae* to trimethoprim resistance.

The usual location of plasmid-borne foreign trimethoprim resistance genes (see later in the chapter) on the chromosome of *C. jejuni* could in a way be classified as chromosomal resistance. In a survey of clinical isolates of this pathogen, it was found that a majority of them carried foreign genes expressing trimethoprim-resistant variations of dihydrofolate reductase. The genes found, *dfr*1 and *dfr*9, are well known as integron- and transposon-borne genes mediating trimethoprim resistance via plasmids in gram-negative enterobacteria. Remnants of the transposon known to carry *dfr*9 were observed in its context on the *Campylobacter* chromosome, and the *dfr*1 was found as an integron cassette (see Chapter 10). The occurrence of these genes could, of course, mediate a very high resistance to trimethoprim, but as mentioned earlier, it is known that *C. jejuni* is intrinsically resistant to this drug by its different enzymatic mechanism for thymidylate synthesis, obviating the need for dihydrofolate reductase, the gene for which, *fol*A, is not to be found on the chromosome of this bacterium. The selective value of acquiring the resistance gene *dfr*1 or *dfr*9 (in some isolates, both were found) is then difficult to understand. Speculatively, for a better growth potential, *C. jejuni* could take advantage of the *dfr* genes, available through antibacterial selection, by complementing its genome, making it able to express a dihydrofolate reductase.

A different type of chromosomal mutation leads to low trimethoprim resistance. Mutations in the *thy*A gene, expressing the enzyme thymidylate synthase, make cells of *E. coli* able to grow in the presence of trimethoprim at concentrations of 8 to 10 μg/mL, provided that there is an external supply of thymine in the medium. The MIC of trimethoprim for *E. coli* is usually just a fraction of a microgram per milliliter. The inactivated thymidylate synthase makes cells dependent on external thymine, but also relieves dihydrofolate reductase of its main task of regenerating tetrahydrofolate in the formation of N^5, N^{10}-methylene tetrahydrofolate, which is oxidized in the deoxyuridylate methylation process (Fig. 3.6). The cell can then afford to have a fraction of its dihydrofolate reductase inactivated by trimethoprim. To turn it around, these low concentrations of trimethoprim could be used for the selection of spontaneous *thy*A mutants if thymine is supplied in the growth medium.

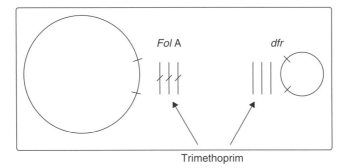

FIGURE 3.7 Plasmid-borne resistance to trimethoprim. Stylized illustration of a gram-negative enterobacterium with its large circular chromosome with the gene for dihydrofolate reductase, *fol*A. The depicted plasmid carries a gene, *dfr*, expressing a trimethoprim-resistant dihydrofolate reductase rescuing the host for survival when the chromosomal dihydrofolate reductase is inactivated by trimethoprim.

Plasmid-Borne Resistance to Trimethoprim

As mentioned earlier, resistance against trimethoprim is presently common and is increasing in frequency. The most common type of trimethoprim resistance in gram-negative enterobacteria (common pathogens of the urinary tract) is represented by foreign genes expressing trimethoprim-resistant dihydrofolate reductases that have been able to transfer themselves horizontally, borne on a transferable plasmid, into the bacterium to make it resistant (Fig. 3.7). These bacteria can then be looked upon as a diploid, of sorts, for *fol*A: that is, the chromosomal gene expressing dihydrofolate reductase in bacteria. The bacterium then becomes resistant since the foreign and resistant dihydrofolate reductase can supply the life-supporting reduction of dihydrofolate to tetrahydrofolate while the normal chromosomal enzyme is inactivated by trimethoprim.

The first of these resistance-mediating genes were found decades ago, but newly found genes seem to be added to the list continuously, where 30 different resistance genes of this type are now to be found. The origin is not known for any one of these genes, but it could be surmised that they come from organisms whose dihydrofolate reductases, by a biological coincidence, have no affinity for trimethoprim. These resistance genes must have moved horizontally into pathogenic bacteria selected by the heavy use of trimethoprim in human medicine and also in veterinary practice. This mechanism, with an extra resistance-mediating target enzyme, is highly prevalent in enterobacteria, where *dfr*1, the first one found, seems to be the most common. It occurs in a cassette in several types of integrons (see Chapter 10). One of these is, in turn, borne on transposon Tn7, which has spread very successfully, mainly because of its high-frequency insertion into a preferred site on the chromosome of *E. coli* and of many other enterobacteria. Among the horizontally moving trimethoprim resistance genes there is a subclass of five genes, *dfr*2a, *dfr*2b, *dfr*2c, *dfr*2d, and *dfr*2e, which are closely related among themselves, but so different from other trimethoprim resistance genes that they cannot be included in the phylogenetic tree, where the interrelationship between the others could be demonstrated (Fig. 3.8).

Their corresponding polypeptides consist of 78 amino acids, and they are 67% identical among the five known enzymes and are active in the form of tetramers showing dihydrofolate reductase activity, which is almost insensitive to trimethoprim, making the host bacterium so resistant that the MIC value cannot be determined, for solubility reasons. Colonies of bacteria carrying these genes can be seen to grow among crystals of trimethoprim on agar plates saturated with the drug. The conspicuous difference from other known dihydrofolate reductases, and their poor enzymic performance (high K_m values and low turnover numbers), make their origin puzzling. Speculatively, it could be surmised that they have another function in their organisms of origin.

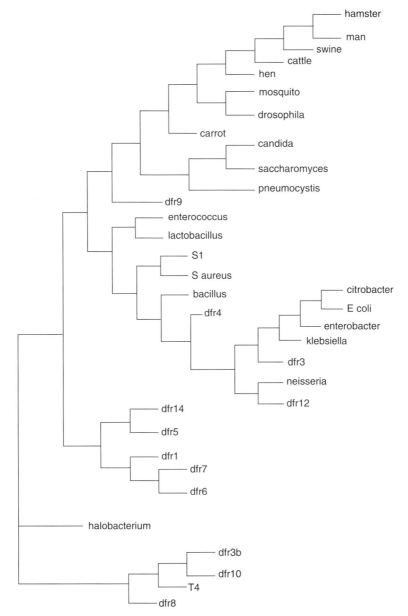

FIGURE 3.8 Phylogenetic tree showing the molecular relationship between dihydrofolate reductases. The relationship was based on amino acid sequences between 35 different dihydrofolate reductases. The resistance dihydrofolate reductases are denoted by *dfr* and a number.

From the phylogenetic tree shown in Figure 3.8 describing the relationship among 35 different dihydrofolate reductases, it can be seen that the resistance enzymes are widely scattered in their relationship with the corresponding enzymes from many organisms. A group of five (*dfr*1, *dfr*5, *dfr*6, *dfr*7, and *dfr*14) with a closer relationship among themselves could be discerned, however. The widely scattered resistance enzymes in the tree, which demonstrate their diversity, are consistent with the notion that these genes have their origins in a large variety of organisms. One, however, *dfr*3, is rather closely related to the chromosomal dihydrofolate reductase of enterobacteria, which could hint at its origin. In staphylococci, extrachromosomally mediated high-level resistance to trimethoprim is effected by the drug-insensitive dihydrofolate reductase S1, borne on the ubiquitously occurring transposon Tn4003. This trimethoprim-resistant enzyme is almost identical to the chromosomal dihydrofolate reductase of *Staphylococcus epidermidis*. It differs by only three amino acid substitutions, and it has therefore been suggested that a mutated form of the *S. epidermidis* enzyme has moved horizontally into other staphylococcal species. A second and similar trimethoprim-resistant and plasmid-encoded dihydrofolate reductase was later isolated from *Staphylococcus haemolyticus*. Its similarity with other staphylococcal enzymes indicated that its origin is similar to that of S1. The S2 enzyme was later found also in *Listeria monocytogenes*.

One of the resistance enzymes of the upper part of the phylogenetic tree, *dfr*9, only distantly related to the main group (Fig. 3.8), was originally found expressed from *dfr*9 on large transferable plasmids in isolates of *E. coli* from swine. The *dfr*9 was observed at a frequency of 11% among these trimethoprim-resistant veterinary isolates of *E. coli* but only very rarely among corresponding human isolates. The spread of *dfr*9 among swine bacteria is probably due to the frequent veterinarian prescription of trimethoprim in swine rearing. A subsequent spread into human commensals might then have taken place. The trimethoprim resistance gene *dfr*9 has been found in patient urinary tract pathogens, although in very few cases. The mechanism of resistance toward trimethoprim described here illustrates the power of the selection pressure exerted by the wide and ubiquitous spread of antibiotics: a power that can force resistance genes to travel horizontally into the pathogens of those infections we try to treat. The horizontal resistance gene transport is effected by genetic transport mechanisms such as plasmids, transposons, and integrons (see Chapter 10), earlier evolved, probably for adaptation to changes in the environment, and now, in turn, used for adaption to the dramatic environmental changes that our use of antibiotics has led to. There is a hint of the origin of the resistance gene *dfr*9 in the upper part of the phylogenetic tree. As mentioned, this gene was found on large transferable plasmids in isolates of *E. coli* from swine. A closer study of the gene environment on the plasmid showed it to be inserted in a crippled transposon, which could be identified as Tn5393, which was crippled because only the right-hand part could be found in the plasmids (Fig. 3.9).

The transposon Tn5393 was originally found and characterized from a plasmid in the plant pathogen *Erwinia amylovora*, causing fire blight in apple trees. It was originally isolated from apple orchards in Michigan. This pathogen caused large losses to fruit farmers, who tried to protect their crops by spraying their apple trees with a solution of streptomycin. The pathogen soon became resistant, however, by taking up two streptomycin resistance genes, *str*A and *str*B (mediating phosphorylation of streptomycin, see Chapter 6). A closer characterization of the resistance showed the two genes to be inserted in a transposon termed Tn5393, which in turn was borne on a plasmid in *E. amylovora*. The right part of Tn5393 was now, as mentioned,

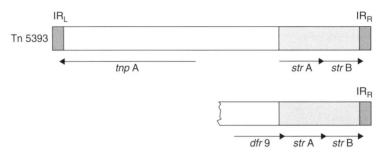

FIGURE 3.9 Transposon Tn5393. Schematic demonstration of the transposon Tn5393 with its transposase gene and its two genes, *str*A and *str*B, for streptomycin resistance and its inverted repeats IRs (see Chapter 10). The lower part of the figure shows the insertion of *dfr*9 in *str*A of the right end of Tn5393 as found on a plasmid in an isolate of *E coli* from swine (see the text).

found on plasmids in the trimethoprim-resistant isolates of *E. coli* from swine and with the resistance-mediating *dfr*9 inserted in the first of the two streptomycin resistance genes, *str*A (Fig. 3.9). The link between *dfr*9, Tn5393, and the further horizontal transport into *E. coli* has not been elucidated, but it illustrates how selection pressure can force resistance genes to pass over long biological distances. That is, a genetic element from a plant pathogen is shown to carry trimethoprim resistance in a gut isolate from swine on another continent. The power of selection is further illustrated in these observations. Modern swine rearing includes herds of hundreds of animals which share gut bacteria. This, in turn, means the existence of enormous populations of genetically communicating bacteria, from which also very rare genetic events can be selected. In this case a gene for trimethoprim resistance borne on a rare movable genetic element could have surfaced under the selection pressure of trimethoprim, which has frequently been used for the treatment of swine diarrhoeas. This might also be an example of how antibiotic resistance genes are brought forward in farm animals, later to find their way into human pathogens. This could very well be the case with *dfr*9, which, as mentioned, has been found in human urinary tract pathogens.

All these examples show bacterial adaptation to the environmental change induced by the ubiquitous use of trimethoprim and by acquiring a large number of different resistance genes, probably originating in a large variation of other organisms. There is a corresponding mechanism of resistance against trimethoprim in staphylococci. This is effected by the transposon-borne and trimethoprim-resistant dihydrofolate reductase S1. In this case the origin of the resistance gene is clear. The resistance enzyme is almost identical to the chromosomal dihydrofolate reductase of *S. epidermidis*. It differs only by three amino acids. It thus seems as if a mutated trimethoprim-resistant form of the enzyme from *S. epidermidis* has spread horizontally into other staphylococcal species. Another plasmid-borne resistance enzyme, S2, mediating trimethoprim resistance horizontally, was observed in *S. haemolyticus* and later also in *L. monocytogenes*. Its structural similarity to S1 indicated a common origin.

Possible Pathogenicity Change in *C. jejuni* by Acquiring Trimethoprim Resistance Genes

It was earlier mentioned that the human pathogen *C. jejuni* is not susceptible to trimethoprim. This innate resistance is explained by the lack of drug target. There is no gene for dihydrofolate reductase on the chromosome of this bacterium. As mentioned earlier, closer studies of the chromosome in clinical isolates of *C. jejuni* showed the occurrence of *dfr*1 and *dfr*9 (i.e., the movable trimethoprim resistance genes found in enterobacteria; see the phylogenetic tree in Fig. 3.8). The mechanisms of horizontal uptake of these genes in *Campylobacter* could be surmised, since they were found inserted in those genetic elements they were earlier found to be used for transfer. In the case of *dfr*1, the gene was found in the characteristic cassette of the integron (see Chapter 10). Regarding *dfr*9, remnants of its earlier Tn5393 surroundings were observed around it. The interpretation of these findings seems to lead to a contradiction, since the trimethoprim resistance genes acquired do not offer any advantage for survival in the presence of trimethoprim. As mentioned earlier, *Campylobacter* bacteria lack a gene for dihydrofolate reductase and are thus innately resistant to trimethoprim. A very speculative, but intriguing interpretation is based on the fact that in the absence of tetrahydrofolate, which in other bacteria is formed by the action of dihydrofolate reductase, the *Campylobacter* use flavonucleotides as reductants in the life-supporting formation of DNA-thymine. Could it be that the lack of a chromosomal gene for dihydrofolate reductase represents an evolutionarily older and less efficient metabolic pattern? The trimethoprim resistance dihydrofolate reductases mobilized by our use of trimethoprim and acquired by *Campylobacter* could possibly enhance the viability of these bacteria, and with that, their pathogenity. Again, this is speculation without experimental support. It ought to be added that either *dfr*1 or *dfr*9 or both presently seem to occur in most or all clinical isolates of *C. jejuni*. Also, *C. jejuni* is a commensal bacterium in the swine gut.

Experimental Test of the Reversibility of Trimethoprim Resistance

In the laboratory experiment of isolating spontaneous sulfonamide-resistant mutants of *E. coli* described earlier in this chapter, a clear fitness cost of resistance could be seen in that the mutationally changed resistance enzyme, the sulfonamide target, dihydropteroate synthase, showed an increased K_m value, that is, was less efficient. This trade-off between resistance and fitness seems to be a logical outcome when a bacterium adapts its evolutionary optimized genotype to one acutely needed in the presence of an antibiotic. On the other hand, as described above, the properties of clinical isolates of N. *meningitidis* seemed to show that resistant strains were not selected against in the absence of sulfonamide. The very important question of possible reversion of resistance should antibiotic use be discontinued or reduced was tested experimentally in a large clinical experiment in a county (Kronoberg) in Sweden. This is a rural part of the country with a population of 178,000. The health care system is funded at the county level and includes two hospitals and 25 primary health care centers. All 464 physicians in the area were asked to substitute trimethoprim-containing medicines with other antibacterials in the treatment of urinary tract infections. This experiment or drug intervention study was performed over 24 months. A prompt and sustained decrease of 85% in the total trimethoprim prescription was reached rapidly, as judged from the sales figures of the distributor. There was, however, no significant trend break in the trimethoprim resistance rate in consecutive isolates of E. *coli*. This apparent lack of effect of the intervention on trimethoprim resistance could be explained by the lack of fitness cost, combined with co-selection by plasmid-associated resistance genes. These results indicate that the cyclic use of antibiotics will not be a useful method for curbing antibiotic resistance development.

CONCLUSION

Sulfonamides and trimethoprim are simple and inexpensive antibacterial agents. Their mechanisms of action are well known and defined at the molecular level. They work by a selective and competitive inhibition of life-supporting enzymes in bacteria. The use of sulfonamides is now very low, mainly because of allergic side effects, whereas trimethoprim is used widely, although its effect is also threatened increasingly by resistance. Sulfonamides might be forced back into clinical use by the general increase in antibiotic resistance, and then with a better understanding and vigilance regarding the allergic side effects. A large part of this chapter has covered sulfonamides, particularly bacterial resistance to them, despite their limited clinical importance today. The purpose of this is to use them as examples, since their mode of action and their mechanisms of resistance are so well known at the molecular level. They could then serve as good examples of evolutionary bacterial adaptation to the environmental change that our use of antibiotics has meant to the microbial world. A better understanding of resistance mechanisms could lead to ways of at least slowing down future resistance development.

CHAPTER 4

PENICILLINS AND OTHER BETALACTAMS

The betalactams, including the penicillins, comprise a large group of antibacterial agents. Microbiological characteristics of beta-lactams, and in what ways their effects suffer from bacterial resistance, are described in this chapter.

The poisonous butterfly sent by the devil is the threatening literary symbol of the prostitute who infects Adrian Leverkühn, the principal character in Thomas Mann's famous novel *Doktor Faustus*, with syphilis. At the end of the novel the death of Leverkühn in the grim and relentless late symptoms of the disease is described. Today, those late symptoms of syphilis are unknown, and most doctors have not even seen a syphilis patient. The bacterial disease syphilis, caused by *T. pallidum*, still exists, but rarely in the Western world, and then in socially isolated circles. In these few cases today it would be a form of malpractice to allow the disease to reach further than to its secondary stage because of a failing diagnosis. In its infectious stage, syphilis is now treatable with a few doses of penicillin, and antimicrobial resistance has not yet emerged. The disease of syphilis could

Antibiotics and Antibiotics Resistance, First Edition. Ola Sköld.
© 2011 John Wiley & Sons, Inc. Published 2011 by John Wiley & Sons, Inc.

in fact serve as a good illustration of the dramatic effect that antibiotics have had on our general health standard. There are ample examples of the scare that the syphilis disease caused among people, as reflected in the world literature. Besides *Doktor Faustus*, there is a stark and dramatic description of the final stages of the disease in Henrik Ibsen's play *Ghosts*. As mentioned, syphilis is a rare disease today, thanks to inexpensive diagnosis with widely available blood tests followed by efficient treatment. The present rarity of the disease means that it can easily be overlooked. This is illustrated by a rather recent case of an elderly man who consulted an ophtalmologist because of increasingly poor eyesight. Examination showed inflammation in the iris area of both eyes, and anti-inflammatory treatment was instituted, despite which eyesight worsened almost to complete blindness. A thorough investigation finally revealed syphilis infection. Penicillin treatment quickly healed the eye inflammation and eyesight was restored almost to normal. The elderly patient was married, but it turned out that in later years he had had sexual contacts with men at summer resorts.

Actually, syphilis meets all of the basic requirements for a disease susceptible to elimination. Humans are the only host; there is no animal reservoir. Also, the complete genome sequence of *Treponema pallidum*, the syphilis spirochete, has been determined, which has revealed clues to what could be developed in a vaccine against the disease.

THE BETALACTAM RING: THE CHARACTERISTIC OF ALL BETALACTAMS

Penicillin was the first antibiotic in a true sense, that is, with its origin in living cells. It was discovered in 1928 but was not used as a remedy until the early 1940s, however (Chapter 1). Its clinical use then resulted immediately in spectacular success, for example, in the treatment of streptococcal infections. The great success induced an intensive interest in the structure of the penicillin molecule and in its antibacterial effect. Early microscopical studies of the effect of penicillin on growing staphylococci showed the bacterial cells as swelling and seeming to explode under the effect of the drug (Fig. 4.1).

If, on the other hand, cells that were not growing because of lack of nutrients were exposed to penicillin (**4-1**), they were unhurt by the drug, since if the penicillin was removed by filtration or centrifugation, and nutrients were added, growth resumed. Penicillin could interfere only with growing bacteria. This, in turn, was interpreted to mean that the penicillin interfered with synthesis of the bacterial cell wall, which, for example,

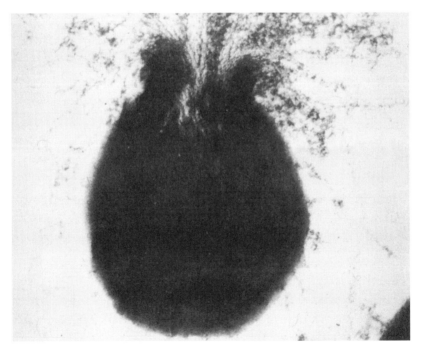

FIGURE 4.1   Effect of penicillin on growing bacterial cells. Microscopical picture of a staphylococcus under the influence of penicillin.

Penicillin G

4-1

protects the integrity of the bacterial cell from internal osmotic pressure in a hypotonic surrounding. It soon turned out that the four-membered cyclic amide with its betalactam bond was the active component of the penicillin molecule, as of all betalactams. If the betalactam bond is severed, the antibacterial effect is lost.

Intensive research and rapidly increasing knowledge of the penicillin molecule soon led to the finding and production of a great number of clinically useful betalactams. Some of these were synthesized in the laboratory, and some were found in living organisms. Figure 1.4 shows a tree of penicillins with many branches representing derivatives of penicillin, all with their origin in the mold *Penicillium chrysogenum* (which is a better producer of penicillin than the original *P. notatum*, identified by Alexander Fleming) and then modified by medicinal chemists to derivatives that could be called *semisynthetic penicillins*. The versatility of penicillins was advanced by the development of a method for modification of the penicillin molecule. Bacterial enzymes were found that could be arranged in a bioreactor to remove the benzyl side chain from penicillin G, leaving 6-aminopenicillanic acid (**4-2**), which could be isolated and then acylated by chemical means. This opened the way to the production of an almost unlimited number of penicillin derivatives. Two groups of betalactams other than penicillins have been found, cephalosporins and monobactams, with their origins in molds and soil bacteria (Fig. 1.4).

6-Aminopenicillanic acid

4-2

The Antibacterial Mechanism of Betalactams

The four-membered betalactam ring is a common feature of all betalactams and a condition for their antibacterial effect, which is directed toward the synthesis of the bacterial cell wall. The cell wall is a common basic entity of virtually all bacteria, and its structure is described in the early chapters of all textbooks of microbiology. The bacterial cell wall is built of long polysaccharide chains that form a backbone of alternating N-acetylglucosamine and its lactyl derivative. These backbone polysaccharide chains are cross-linked between themselves by peptides to form the structure called *peptidoglycan*. It can be looked at as a giant molecule structured as an armor enveloping the bacterium and protecting it against, for example, osmotic lysis. The stability of the cell wall depends on the peptide cross-links. These are formed by a sequence of known biochemical reactions, where a pentapeptide linked to a monosaccharide and containing a diaminoamino acid (lysine or diaminopimelic acid) with two D-alanins at the end is transported out through the cell membrane to that energyless world outside the cell membrane of the bacterial cell, where the cell wall is formed. The monosaccharide is incorporated in a growing polysaccharide chain of the cell wall, and the carboxyl group at the end of the peptide can form a peptide bond with the diaminoamino acid of an incorporated peptide of a neighboring polysaccharide chain, thus forming a covalent link between two polysaccharide chains.

The cross-linking peptide bond is formed in an energy-less environment and is effected by a transpeptidation reaction, where one of the two D-alanins at the end of the incoming peptide chain is split off and transfers its peptide bond to the free amino group of the diaminoamino acid of a nearby peptide of the growing cell wall. This transpeptidation reaction is catalyzed by a membrane-bound transpeptidase enzyme, which is a penicillin-binding protein, described further later in the chapter. The betalactams inhibit this transpeptidation reaction by a structural analogy between the betalactam ring and the D-alanyl-D-alanine dipeptide at the end of the cross-linking peptide. Inhibition of the transpeptidation inhibits the cross-linking in cell wall formation making the newly formed cell wall unstable. This is well illustrated by the bacteriolysis that can be observed in a test tube culture of for example staphylococci after the addition of a small amount (a few tenths of a microgram per milliliter) of penicillin (Fig. 4.1). It follows from this argument that only growing bacterial cells are affected by betalactams, since only the formation of cross-links is interfered with. Nongrowing bacterial cells are completely unaffected by the presence of betalactams.

PENICILLINS

The first penicillin isolated, penicillin G, or benzylpenicillin (**4-1**) is still used to a large extent. It has to be administered parenterally, however, since it is acid labile and will be destroyed by stomach acidity. A simple remodelling of the molecule to phenoxymethylpenicillin, penicillin V (**4-3**), results in acid stability and so in a penicillin that resists the acidity of the stomach and can be given per os. Penicillins G and V both have a narrow antibacterial spectrum, which means that their effect is directed primarily against a limited number of bacteria, mostly gram-positive cocci, whereas gram-negative enterobacteria are

Phenoximethyl penicillin

4-3

unaffected at corresponding doses. Supposedly, this is due to the thick outer lipopolysaccharide layer of gram-negative bacteria, which penicillins G and V cannot easily penetrate.

Penicillins with an Enlarged Spectrum

A simple change in the side chain of penicillins leading to ampicillin (**4-4**) mediates a much higher activity against gram-negative bacteria, but at the cost of its activity against gram-positive cocci. The antibacterial spectrum of ampicillin has been moved toward the gram-negative side, which means that ampicillin cannot be called a broad-spectrum penicillin. Ampicillin is acid stable and shows a variable uptake from the gastrointestinal tract, which means that it can interfere with the normal composition of the mostly gram-negative commensal bacteria of the gut and cause enteritis symptoms. Another small change in the penicillin side chain, the addition of a hydroxyl group, results in amoxycillin (**4-5**), which is rapidly absorbed from the gastrointestinal tract almost completely, then without interfering with the normal bacterial composition in the colon. The pivampicillin (**4-6**) and bacampicillin (**4-7**) penicillin derivatives, which also have a good effect against gram-negative bacteria, were synthesized with the same goal of rapid and complete uptake from the gastrointestinal tract. The principle is different, however. Both pivampicillin and bacampillin are prodrugs with structural side groups that allow them to be absorbed rapidly at the upper part of the

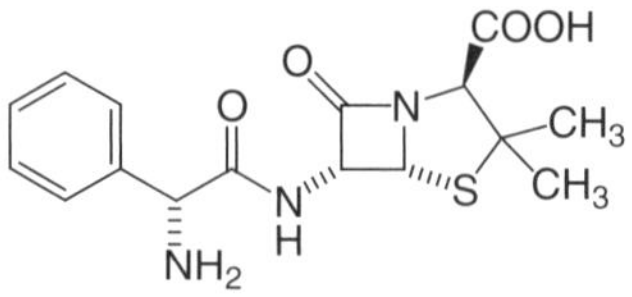

Ampicillin

4-4

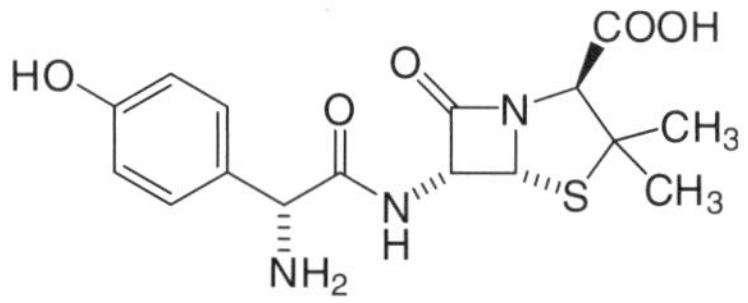

Amoxycillin

4-5

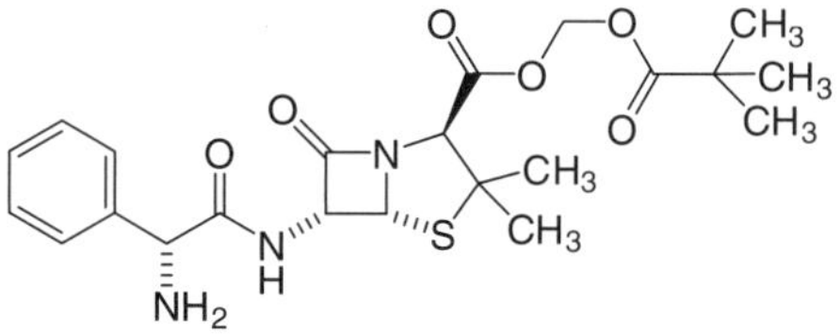

Pivampicillin

4-6

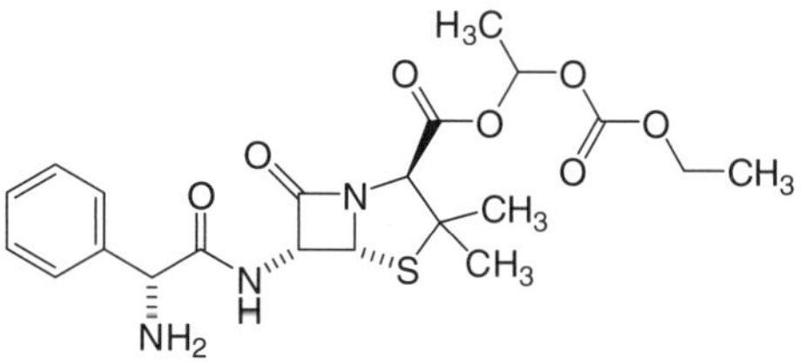

Bacampicillin

4-7

gastrointestinal tract, where on passing the mucous membrane their side groups are split off to yield ampicillin.

In mecillinam, the side chain is attached differently to the penicillin nucleus. It is also effective primarily against gram-negative rods, much less so against gram-positive cocci. Mecillinam also seems to have a different mechanism of action, not inhibiting the transpeptidation at the cell wall formation, but binding to another penicillin-binding protein (PBP2) involved in the reorganization of the cell wall in gram-negative bacteria. The cell wall peptidoglycan can be regarded as a covalently bound giant molecule enclosing the cell. For the cell to be able to grow and divide, this armor must be plastic and be able to reorganize its structure. Bacterial cells affected by mecillinam show abnormal egglike structures when looked at under the microscope.

Penicillins Stable to Penicillinases

The most common form of bacterial resistance against betalactams is that the pathogenic bacterium produces a betalactamase, an enzyme cleaving the betalactam bond and thus inactivating the ability of the betalactam to interfere with the bacterial cell wall synthesis. The first observations of penillin inactivation by betalactamase, or penicillinase, as it was then called, were made in staphylococci at the end of the 1940s. The betalactamase hydrolyzes the betalactam bond of the penicillin with penicilloic acid (**4-8**) as a product. More than 90% of nosocomial *Staphylococcus aureus* isolates today are penicillin resistant because of an acquired betalactamase.

Penicilloic acid

4-8

These early observations of penicillin inactivation led to ideas about protecting the betalactam bond by chemical manipulation of the side chain to keep the betalactamase away and obtain penicillins stable to penicillinases. The first derivative synthesized along these lines was methicillin (**4-9**), in its side chain carrying large and bulky methoxy groups, which were thought to reach over the betalactam bond to protect it. Methicillin did turn out to be a poor substrate for the staphylococcal penicillinase, which was found to degrade methicillin 30 times slower than it degraded penicillin G (benzylpenicillin). Methicillin has little effect on gram-negative bacteria and is acid labile, which means that it has to be administered parenterally. Its present clinical use is very low. Its name is frequently used, however, in the feared form of clinical resistance, methicillin-resistant *Staphylococcus aureus* (MRSA), which expresses itself as clones of staphylococci resistant to all betalactams and spreading epidemically. This resistance of MRSA is not caused by betalactamase but by a horizontally mediated uptake of a foreign gene expressing a penicillin-binding protein (PBP2a) with a very low affinity for all betalactams. This is described later in the chapter in more detail.

Methicillin

4-9

The further search for betalactam varieties in which the betalactam bond was protected from betalactamases led to the isoxazolyl penicillins (oxacillins; **4-10**), where a large and bulky isoxazolyl group in the side chain was thought to obstruct the betalactamases from attacking the betalactam bond. This interpretation was later modified to regard the penicillinase

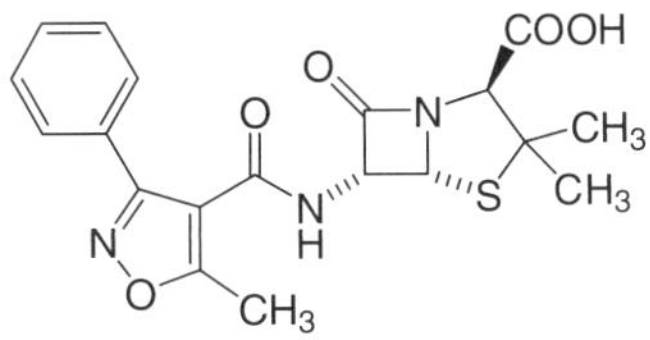

Oxacillin

4-10

stability of these modified betalactams as being due to a variable substrate specificity among betalactamases, (see our discussion of betalactamases later in the chapter). It turned out that different betalactamases showed very different substrate spectra. The staphylococcal betalactamase simply does not recognize isoxazolyl penicillin as a substrate. Other betalactamases with different substrate profiles, which include isoxazolyl penicillin, were found later, however. So many betalactamases are now known that for all betalactams used clinically, one or several betalactamases have been found attacking it; that is, the substrate profiles of these enzymes are so varied that all known betalactams are included in them.

Cloxacillin (**4-11**), dicloxacillin (**4-12**), and flukloxacillin (**4-13**) also belong to the isoxazolyl penicillins. They differ by carrying different chlorine and fluorine substitutions in the side chain which have been introduced for pharmacokinetic reasons. They have found use in the treatment of staphylococcal bone infections. MRSA strains, are also resistant to isoxazolyl penicillins.

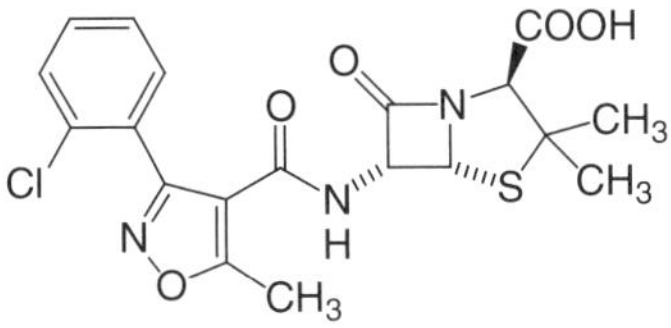

Cloxacillin

4-11

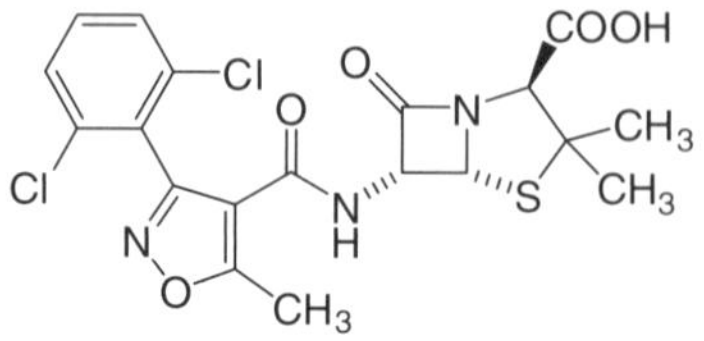

Dicloxacillin

4-12

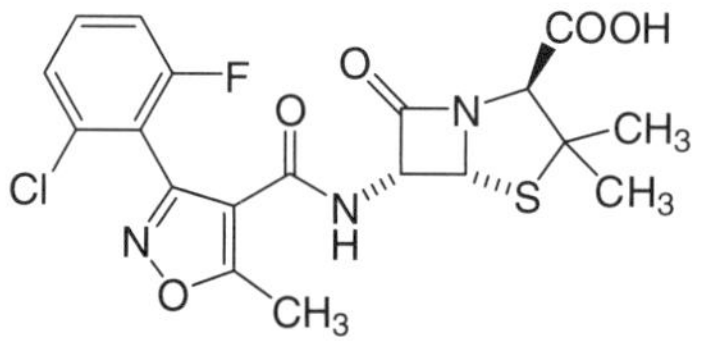

Flucloxacillin

4-13

Counteracting Resistance by the Inhibition of Betalactamases

Clavulanic acid (**4-14**) is an uncharacteristic betalactam (Fig. 1.4) that has a five-membered heterocyclic, oxygen-containing ring structure attached to the betalactam structure instead of the typical sulfur-containing ring (thiazolidin) of penicillins. The antibacterial effect of this betalactam is too weak for clinical use as an antibacterial drug. It has, however, another property that makes it useful in the context of treating bacterial infections with penicillins. When attacked by a betalactamase, its betalactam bond is hydrolyzed as with other betalactams, but this reaction leads to an irreversible inactivation of the enzyme. That is, the betalactamase commits suicide by exposing its active center to a covalent binding with the hydrolysis product of clavulanic acid. There are two other such suicide inhibitors, sulbactam and tazobactam, which are more similar to penicillin in that they have five-membered sulfur-containing rings attached to the betalactam structure. The sulfur in these rings is

Clavulanic acid
4-14

oxidized to a sulfone. This inhibition phenomenon has been turned to advantage by combining clavulanic acid with a penicillin such as amoxycillin. The combination is then efficient against betalactamase-producing pathogens. The betalactamase inactivation by clavulanic acid protects the penicillin from enzymic degradation.

Very soon, however, resistance against this combination was also observed. The TEM betalactamase (see later in the chapter) production in enterobacteria could, for example, increase to hyperproduction by mutations in the regulatory mechanism. Also, mutations could induce various amino acid changes in the TEM betalactamase to produce inhibitor-resistant TEM derivatives, decreasing their binding affinity to clavulanic acid, which is then excluded from their substrate profile. The destructive effect of clavulanic acid on the betalactamase cannot take place, and in turn its protecting effect on the penicillin is abolished (Fig. 4.2). These mutationally changed betalactamases retain their betalactam-cleaving ability but have become refractory to clavulanic acid.

OTHER ANTIBACTERIAL BETALACTAMS

Cephalosporins

Cephalosporins and penicillins are closely related, but cephalosporins were isolated from another group of microorganisms, *Cephalosporium*. Cephalosporins differ from penicillins

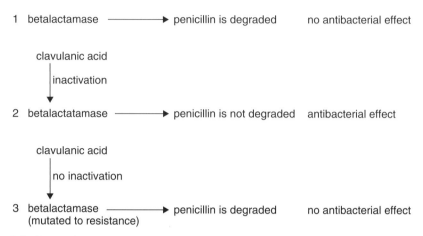

FIGURE 4.2 Effect of clavulanic acid in protecting penicillin against resistance: the protecting effect of clavulanic acid against the degradation of penicillin by betalactamase, and neutralization of the protecting effect by mutational changes in the substrate specificity of the betalactamase. In example 1, penicillin is degraded by betalactamase to destroy its antibacterial effect; in example 2, the presence of clavulanic acid protects penicillin by inactivating the betalactamase present in the infecting bacterium, and the antibacterial effect is intact; in example 3, the infecting bacterium possesses a betalactamase that has mutated to exclude clavulanic acid from its substrate spectrum to make it resistant against its inhibiting effect, and the betalactamase present will then destroy the antibacterial effect of penicillin.

by having a six-membered, heterocyclic, sulfur-containing ring (dihydrothiazine) attached to the four-membered betalactam ring. The first cephalosporin isolated from *Cephfalosporium* was cephalosporin C (**4-15**), of which many semisynthetic derivatives were later produced, showing differences in antibacterial spectra and in susceptibilities to different betalactamases. In analogy with penicillin G, the side chain of cephalosporin C can be removed enzymically to give 7-aminocephalosporanic acid, which can be acylated chemically to give new derivatives.

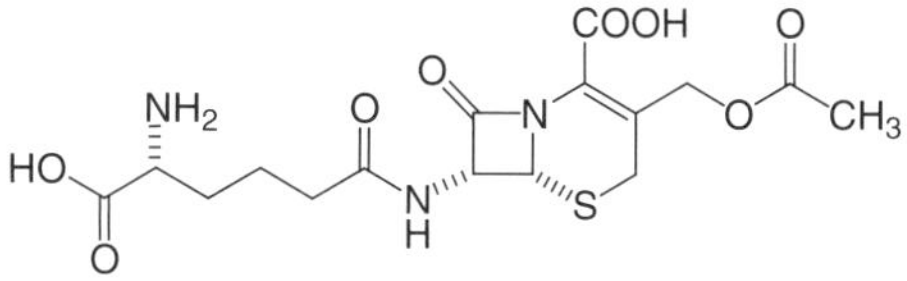

Cephalosporin C

4-15

The first successful semisynthetic cephalosporin was cephaloridine (**4-16**). Many others have followed. Most are effective only when given parenterally, but cephalexin and cefixime can be given per os. Cefuroxime is not degraded by many common betalactamases and can then be used against pathogens that are resistant to many other betalactams. Like all betalactams, cephalosporins work by interfering with the cell wall synthesis of growing bacteria. As indicated, there have been both medical and commercial incentives for medicinal chemists to synthesize cephalosporin modifications. One has been to obtain new betalactams with wide antibacterial spectra embracing different pathogens. Another reason has been to find betalactams with an increased ability to resist betalactamases, which have been observed to increase in frequency among pathogenic bacteria. The latter goal has turned out to be very difficult to achieve, at least for more than a short time, since betalactamase evolution seems to have been able to keep pace with the ability of medicinal chemists to produce new derivatives.

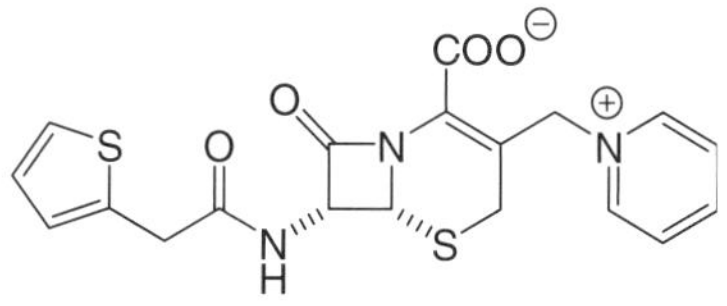

Cephaloridin

4-16

One further specific cephalosporin ought to be mentioned here: ceftobiprole (**4-17**), which is new and is said to belong to the fifth generation of cephalosporin derivatives. It is resistant to *S. aureus* betalactamase and has the important property of binding to and inhibiting the 2a penicillin binding protein of MRSA. See our discussion of MRSA and its treatment with antibacterials later in the chapter. It is also effective against penicillin-resistant *Streptococcus pneumoniae* strains and against penicillin-resistant *Pseudomonas* strains. There is a clinical disadvantage in that it has to be administered intravenously.

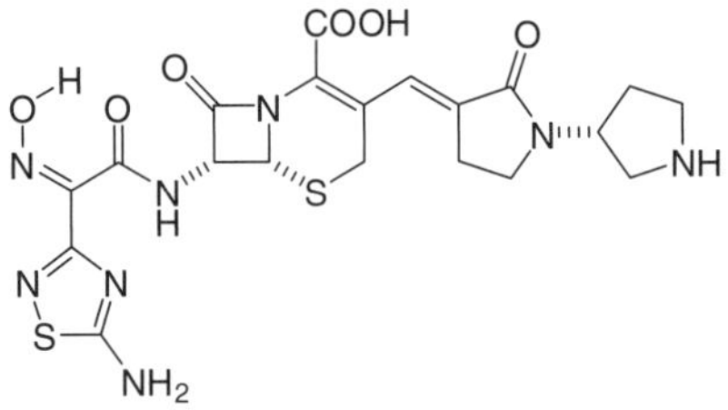

Ceftobiprole

4-17

Monobactams

The medical success of penicillins and cephalosporins led to an intensive search for further betalactams from microorganisms. One finding along these lines was that of monobactams occurring in soil bacteria (Fig. 1.4). In these, the four-membered antibacterial betalactam structure is alone and not fused to another heterocyclic ring as in penicillins and cephalosporins. It represents the simplest betalactam that has an antibacterial effect. One semisynthetic monobactam preparation is aztreonam (**4-18**; trade name, Azactam). It has a good effect on gram-negative bacteria. It was announced as being stable to betalactamases but has been shown to be hydrolyzed by betalactamases with an extended spectrum. (see our discussion of betalactamases later in the chapter).

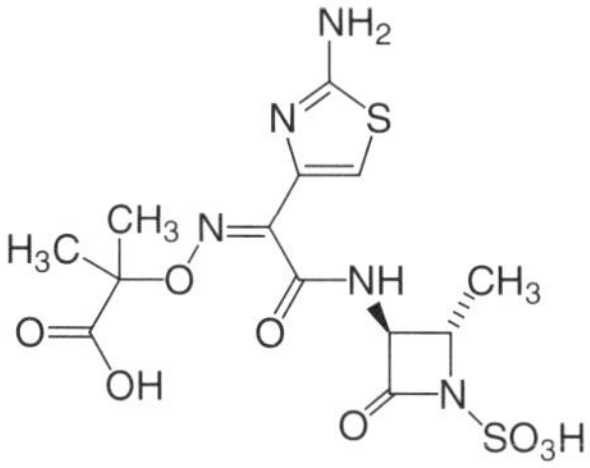

Aztreonam

4-18

Monobactams have an additional clinical benefit related to allergies to penicillin, which some people suffer from. This happens because penicillin binds covalently to a blood protein, which the immune system then recognizes as a foreign protein. The immune system responds to it in the future by mounting an attack on penicillin and many other betalactams, whether or not they are linked to a protein. This attack triggers an usually serious allergic response. People allergic to penicillin as described can be treated safely with monobactams, which do not trigger an allergic response in the way that other betalactams would do.

Thienamycins

Another group of betalactams found in soil bacteria are the thienamycins, the first member of which, thienamycin (**4-19**), was found in *Streptomyces cattleya*. Thienamycins are structurally similar to penicillins but without sulfur in the five-membered ring attached to the betalactam ring; instead, the side chain contains sulfur. This characteristic makes them belong to the larger group of carbapenems. Thienamycins are efficient antibacterials and show a broad antibacterial spectrum. Furthermore, they are remarkably resistant to betalactamases. Thienamycin itself is very labile and decomposes in water solution, so is therefore impractical for clinical use. Imipenem is an *N*-formimidoyl derivative of thienamycin that is used clinically. It can only

Thienamycin

4-19

be administered parenterally and has to be combined vith cilastin, an inhibitor of renal dihydropeptidase, which would otherwise rapidly degrade the imipenem. Meropenem is a further developed semisynthetic derivative of thienamycin, which resists the renal dihydropeptidase and can therefore be administered without the peptidase inhibitor cilastin. Still another thienamycin derivative is ertapenem, which is structurally similar to meropenem.

There is a recently discovered property of meropenem that could make it useful in the increasingly difficult treatment of tuberculosis: difficult because the disease-causing agent *Mycobacterium tuberculosis* has increasingly shown resistance to previously efficient antituberculosis drugs (see Chapter 9), resulting in extensively drug-resistant (XDR) clinical strains of the disease-causing bacterium. Betalactams have never been of much use in the treatment of tuberculosis, and one reason for the lack of efficiency of betalactams in this context was found in the genome sequence of *M. tuberculosis*, which contains a gene for a highly active betalactamase (see below). Laboratory experiments have now shown that meropenem in combination with clavulanic acid (mentioned earlier in the chapter) shows synergistically a strong killing effect on the disease-causing bacterium in its XDR forms also.

It should finally be mentioned here that the long and time-consuming work to develop betalactam antibacterials, mainly to counteract betalactamases, has meant more and more expensive preparations. The defined daily dose of one of the new thien-amycin derivatives is more than 300 times more expensive than the corresponding dose of penicillin V.

BETALACTAMASES

Betalactamases, or penicillinases as they were then called, had been discovered by the end of the 1940s. As mentioned earlier, these enzymes have the ability to hydrolyze the betalactam bond of betalactams to destroy their antibacterial activity completely. The cleavage product of this enzymic reaction with penicillin is penicilloic acid, which lacks antibacterial activity. Today, more than 200 different betalactamases are known. They differ from each other by having different substrate profiles toward penicillins, cephalosporins and monobactams, and carbapenems. They can be classified after their substrate profile, which can include clavulanic acid. Some of the betalactamases do not attack clavulanic acid, since it is not included in their substrate profile; clavulanic acid is simply not recognized by the active center of these enzymes. The oxacillinases also include the isoxazolyl derivatives cloxacillin, dicloxacillin, and flucloxacillin among their substrates, mediating resistance to these penicillin deriva-tives, originally marketed as penicillinase-stable penicillins. In later years two groups of betalactamases also hydrolyzing thien-amycins (imipenem, meropenem, ertapenem) have been identi-fied in pathogenic bacteria (carbapenemases). This illustrates the statement that for any clinically used betalactam, a betalactamase has also been found.

Horizontal Spread of Betalactamases

The very widely spread betalactam resistance among pathogenic bacteria is in large part due to the horizontal transfer of betalac-tamase genes from bacterium to bacterium, also promiscuously between related species. The first horizontal transfer of betalactamase activity discovered between bacteria was described in 1963 by Naomi Datta in London and Polyxeni Kontomichalou in Athens. The betalactamase studied by these two bacteriologists became known under the name TEM after the Greek patient (Temoniera) from whom the betalactamase-carrying strain of *E. coli* studied had been isolated. Datta and Kontomichalou could show that the gene expressing the TEM enzyme was borne on a transferable plasmid, which by its conjugation mechanism could transfer itself from bacterium to bacterium.

Among penicillin-resistant bacteria, the TEM enzyme is still the most common cause of resistance. It has a defined substrate spectrum, which is illustrated in Table 4.1, where the two top lines show that the MIC value for ampicillin increases more than 64-fold in an *E. coli* strain carrying TEM (TEM-1) borne on an R plasmid. This means that ampicillin is a good substrate for this betalactamase, which could not at all degrade the cephalosporins cefotaxim, ceftazidim, or cefuroxime and also not the monobactam aztreonam or the carbapenem imipenem. This *E. coli* strain is

TABLE 4.1 Betalactamases of the TEM Type with Their Substrate Spectra Extended by Point Mutations

		MIC (mg/L)[a]					
Bacterium	Betalactamase[b]	Ampicillin	Aztreonam	Cephotaxim	Ceftazidim	Cefuroxim	Imipenem
E. coli	R-	4	0.125	0.125	0.25	8.0	0.25
	TEM-1	>256	0.125	0.125	0.25	8.0	0.25
	TEM-12	>256	8.0	0.5	64.0	8.0	0.25
	TEM-26	>256	32.0	1.0	256.0	16.0	0.25

[a]The substrate spectrum is reflected in the susceptibility of the host carrying the betalactamases, expressed as MIC values (expressed as mg/L) for the betalactams tested.

[b]R- connotes an *E. coli* bacterium not carrying an R plasmid; TEM-1 is the corresponding bacterium with an R plasmid mediating the TEM betalactamase gene. TEM-12 and TEM-26 are mutated forms of TEM-1 (see the text).

thus sensitive to these antibiotics despite its resistance to ampicillin. It has been shown, however, that a mutation, one single DNA base exchange in the enzyme gene, could modify the substrate specificity of the TEM enzyme to change the resistance pattern of the host.

The third line of Table 4.1 shows the changed substrate profile for a mutated TEM-12, where one amino acid close to the active center of the enzyme has been exchanged. A point mutation has effected the substitution of an arginine for a serine. This has changed the substrate profile of the enzyme to include in its substrate spectrum the cephalosporins cefotaxim and ceftazidim and the monobactam aztreonam. One single mutation in the TEM gene thus extends its substrate spectrum markedly and widens the resistance pattern of the host. This is an example of the larger phenomenon of extended spectrum betalactamases (ESBLs), which has become a serious clinical problem in the treatment of bacterial diseases with antibiotics.

The fourth line of Table 4.1 describes the effect of two amino acid changes in TEM to give TEM-26, where in addition to the arginine–serine exchange (TEM-12) there is also a glutamic acid–lysine exchange. These amino acid changes dramatically affect the resistance pattern of the host bacterium, which now retains only its susceptibility to imipenem. Those simple mutational changes have widened the substrate spectrum of the betalactamase and in consequence also widened the pattern of resistance that it can mediate. Many variations of TEM with a widened and increased effect against several betalactams have now been characterized. The clinical phenomenon of ESBLs is an evolutionary consequence of the worldwide and ubiquitous use of betalactams. The work of medicinal chemists to find new betalactams and to modify existing ones has aimed primarily at fighting resistance by finding derivatives outside the substrate spectra of clinically known betalactamases.

Simple mutations resulting in ESBLs could thus destroy millions of research dollars in the pharmaceutical industry.

Penicillin-Binding Proteins

Penicillin-binding proteins (PBPs) are involved in the formation of the cell wall in all bacteria and are the targets of betalactam antibiotics. The colon bacterium *E. coli*, for example, has eight different proteins in this category. PBP1a and PBP1b of these in *E. coli* are responsible for the transpeptidase reaction mentioned earlier in the chapter which forms those cross-links, which are a condition for the stability of the cell wall. These two proteins are membrane bound. Penicillin-binding proteins 2 and 3 in *E. coli* also show transpeptidase activity but seem to be involved in the continuous reorganization of the wall, which has to take place during cell growth. This interpretation is supported by the fact that the betalactam mecillinam binds primarily to PBP2 and induces gram-negative bacteria to form abnormal egglike cells when it acts on growing bacteria. The other PBPs in *E. coli* show carboxypeptidase activity and are involved in the continuous reformation of the cell wall at cell growth. These PBPs seem to be involved in regulating the transpeptidation by the splitting of the peptide bond between the two D-alanins located at the end of the pentapeptide. All PBPs have a highly conserved serine residue in their active site that forms an ester with the carbonyl group at the opened betalactam bond. This serine ester is a structural analog of the normal substrate of the PBP, that is, the D-ala-D-ala at the end of the pentapeptide involved in the transpeptidation reaction leading to those cross-links that are crucial for cell wall stability (as discussed earlier in the chapter). This makes the PBP nonfunctional since the ester with the betalactam is hydrolyzed very slowly in comparison with the natural substrate, D-ala-D-ala. The antibacterial effect of betalactams is dependent on their efficient binding to the PBPs of the bacterial cell. Some bacteria manage to escape this by acquiring PBPs that bind less readily to betalactams and are thus not inactivated by the drug.

Resistance to Betalactams by Changes in the PBPs

As mentioned, a diminished affinity for betalactams to the penicillin-binding proteins (PBPs) is an important form of beta-lactam resistance in bacteria besides the action of betalactamases. The origins of these low-affinity PBPs are very diverse. A good example of this is *Staphylococcus aureus* resistant to methicillin (MRSA). This is a pathogen resistant to practically all betalac-tams, and thus very difficult to treat. *S. aureus* is one of the most successful human pathogens. It is carried by about 30% of the healthy human population on the skin and in the nostrils. Despite its usually benign lifestyle, it has a formidable pathogenic poten-tial. Before the use of antibiotics, 80% of all septicemias caused by it were fatal. The spread of strains resistant to methicillin and other antibiotics is thus a challenging public health prob-lem. MRSA is often spread nosocomially: that is, from patient to patient in hospitals. The methicillin-resistant staphylococci also often show resistance to practically all other antibacterial agents. Vancomycin-resistant MRSA have been identified in several parts of the world. These pathogens seem to be insensitive to all clini-cally available antibacterial agents. The methicillin resistance in MRSA is mediated by the *mec*A gene, which in turn is borne on a large (50-kb) DNA fragment inserted in the staphylococ-cal chromosome. The *mec*A gene expresses a penicillin-binding protein (PBP2′ or PBP2a) with a very low affinity for penicillins, which will take over the corresponding PBP functions of its host and make it resistant to all betalactams. The *mec*A gene must have moved horizontally into *S. aureus* from another bacterial species, and it has been shown that a *mec*A homolog can be found on the chromosome of *Staphylococcus sciuri*, the name of which relates to the Latin name for squirrel, but it has also been isolated from staphylococci of many other rodents. MRSA is, of course, much feared because of the difficulties in treating the infections it causes. It is interesting to compare their frequencies in different areas. In a recent European survey of staphylococcal isolates from hospital intensive-care units, MRSA frequencies varied from 0% in two countries to 60% in six other countries. It has turned out that strict conditions against the spread of the contagion has an effect on MRSA frequencies. All these observations demonstrate the intriguing strategies that bacteria can use to protect themselves from antibiotics by the horizontal transfer of resistance-mediating DNA.

There are other cases of betalactam resistance by the occurrence of PBPs with a lowered affinity for betalactams. The clinically most important of these involve *Streptococcus pneumoniae* pneumococci, causing bacterial pneumonia, otitis, septicemia, and many other diseases. In these pathogens, penicillin resistance is due entirely to alterations in the properties of the PBPs. Pneumococci are important pathogens from an international point of view. Unfortunately, they show a rapid increase in resistance correlated to a large international distribution of betalactams. The level of increased resistance to penicillin is more than 1000-fold. Calculations have shown that within a short time almost half of all pneumococcal isolates at the Centers for Disease Control in Atlanta, Georgia will be penicillin resistant. Also in Scandinavia, penicillin-resistant pneumococci causing clinical problems have occurred at a frequency of 5 to 10%. Betalactam resistance in *S. pneumoniae* has been shown to be caused by stepwise horizontal transfers of DNA, resulting in mosaic genes expressing PBPs with a diminished affinity for betalactams. These changes occur in the transpeptidase domains of the penicillin binding protein PBP2B of *S. pneumoniae*. The gene fragments incorporated have been shown to have their origins in other commensal species of streptococci. The development of PBPs with greatly decreased affinity for betalactams seems to require the introduction of multiple amino acid substitutions in order to rearrange the active center of the enzyme so that it can exclude the antibiotic without impairing its ability to recognize its structurally analogous (D-ala-D-ala) peptide structure in the transpeptidase reaction.

The diminishing affinities of the PBPs of pneumococci to give penicillin resistance seem to have occurred since the introduction of penicillin in the 1940s, and it is an extreme example of the ability of an enzyme to evolve to discriminate between its substrate and a structurally analogous inhibitor, under the intense selective pressure of ubiquitously distributed betalactams. This resistance phenomenon parallels the sulfonamide resistance in *N. meningitidis* described in Chapter 3. In the latter case, resistance is mediated by DNA fragments inserted in the chromosomal gene expressing dihydropteroate synthase, the target enzyme for sulfonamides. Both *Streptococcus* and *Neisseria* have the ability of natural transformation, allowing a spontaneous exchange of DNA between related bacterial cells. Both the middle ear and the nasopharynx can be imagined to provide favorable conditions for the horizontal transfer of DNA between commensal and pathogenic pneumococci, and where recombinants with a lowered susceptibility to betalactams could be selected under the selective pressure of betalactams, used often in the treatment of pneumococcal disease. The recombinants selected have been observed to occur in clones, which have spread epidemically all over the world. They have been identified as, for example, the "Spanish-American" clone and the "French" clone. The epidemic spread of resistance clones could be partially controlled by strict hygiene and patient isolation. Where tested, measures of contagion protection have been shown to be quite effective. This betalactam resistance in *S. pneumoniae* is another example of how bacteria can escape the poisonous effect of our antibiotics by using naturally occurring evolutionary mechanisms.

A VERY OLD PROPHECY CAME TRUE

Penicillins, which are widely distributed, are still a very much appreciated group of antibacterial agents. Close to half of all antibiotic prescriptions in Sweden are for penicillins, which means that almost all citizens have taken penicillin once or several times, mostly in the form of tablets. This intensive—too intensive—use of penicillins and of other betalactams in Sweden and in the world has for decades effected a selection pressure that has caused the now very widespread betalactam resistance among pathogenic bacteria. Alexander Fleming, the discoverer of penicillin, foresaw this. In an interview in the *New York Times* in 1945, he very farsightedly warned that overuse of penicillin could lead to the development of resistant bacteria. In laboratory experiments he had himself observed that bacteria grown in gradually increasing concentrations of penicillin became resistant to penicillin in concentrations comparable to those that could be achieved in blood serum in the antibacterial treatment of patients. In those cases at that time, resistance was caused by mutational changes in the cellular permeability for penicillin. Today, those resistance levels would be regarded as so low that they could be handled by increasing doses. Fleming particularly warned against penicillin that in the future could be taken per os (in 1945, acid-stable fenoxymethyl penicillin was not yet available), which would lead to self-medication with overuse as a consequence together with a following selection of resistant pathogens. These could spread from person to person and cause therapeutic failures. This almost 70-year-old prophecy by Fleming was remarkably precise and has come true to a much larger extent than could be imagined at that time.

CHAPTER 5

GLYCOPEPTIDES

Glycopeptides interfere with bacterial cell wall synthesis, as do the betalactams, but these two groups of antibacterial agents are completely unrelated in terms of their structure and provenance. As do the betalactams, glycopeptides inhibit the transpeptidation reaction (Chapter 4), which is the key reaction in establishing cell wall stability. In the presence of glycopeptides the cell wall becomes unstable, and the bacterial cells affected become prone to lysis. The two glycopeptides used clinically, vancomycin (**5-1**) and teichoplanin (**5-2**), are antibiotics in the true sense (i.e., they were originally found in living organisms). Vancomycin in a soil bacterium, *Streptomyces orientalis*, was observed first in Borneo, but later in soil samples from many other places. Clinical use of vancomycin began in 1958. Vancomycin and teichoplanin are not absorbed when given per os; they have to be administered parenterally. Their principal use is against gram-positive cocci, and they have more or less been reserved for severe infections with multiresistant pathogens, and have tended to be regarded as remedies of last resort: for example, in

Antibiotics and Antibiotics Resistance, First Edition. Ola Sköld.
© 2011 John Wiley & Sons, Inc. Published 2011 by John Wiley & Sons, Inc.

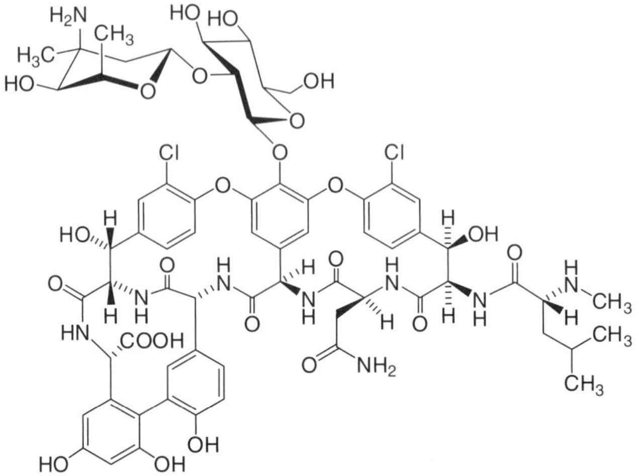

Vancomycin

5-1

the treatment of methicillin-resistant stafylococci (MRSA) and of multiresistant pneumococci causing septicemia and meningitis. The lack of glycopeptide absorbtion from the gastrointestinal canal can be turned into an advantage in infections caused by the toxin-producing anaerobic bacterium *Clostridium difficile*, which can cause life-threatening colitis infections when the normal bacterial composition in the intestine has been disturbed by antibiotic treatment. Vancomycin given in capsules works well against the often life-threatening *Clostridium* colitis.

MECHANISM OF ANTIBACTERIAL ACTION

As mentioned, glycopeptides interfere with the transpeptidation reaction at bacterial cell wall formation, parallel to the action of betalactams. The glycopeptides, however, bind to the D-ala-D-ala end of the peptide, which is the substrate of the transpeptidase reaction cross-linking the polysacharide chains of the cell wall structure (Chapter 4). Glycopeptides do not penetrate the

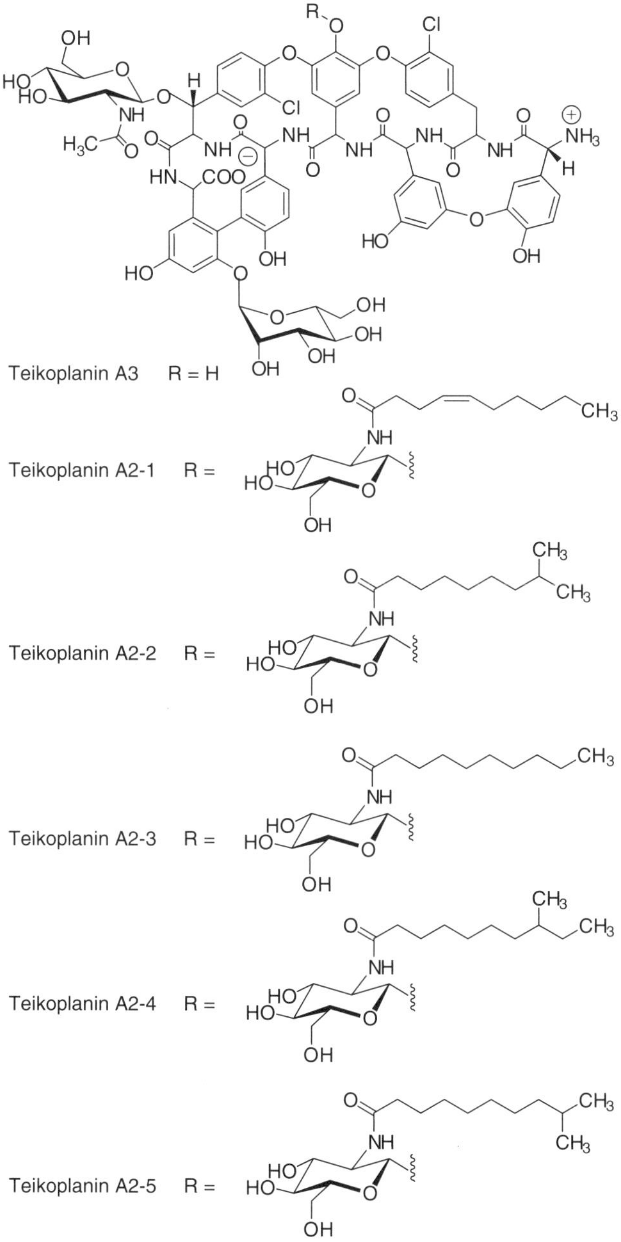

Teikoplanin A3   R = H

Teikoplanin A2-1   R =

Teikoplanin A2-2   R =

Teikoplanin A2-3   R =

Teikoplanin A2-4   R =

Teikoplanin A2-5   R =

Teichoplanin

5-2

cytoplasm, and interaction with the target can only take place when the precursor peptide has been translocated to the outer surface of the cytoplasmic membrane. The large and bulky glycopeptide molecule bound to the two D-alanins at the peptide end inhibits the transpeptidation and, consequently, the cross-linking. The final effect is the same as with the betalactams (i.e., cell wall lability and lysis of bacterial cells).

RESISTANCE

The resistance of gram-positive cocci to glycopeptides (usually, there is cross-resistance between vancomycin and teichoplanin and also with avoparcin, discussed later in the chapter) is caused by a rather complicated series of enzymatic reactions, leading to the substitution of the D-ala at the very end of the cross-linking peptide with a D-lactate residue. The glycopeptide does not recognize its antibacterial target very well when it has changed to D-ala-D-lac (Fig. 5.1). Its affinity for the changed target is, in fact, 1000-fold lower than for the normal D-ala-D-ala structure. The transpeptidation is no longer inhibited by the glycopeptide and can proceed by splitting off the lactate residue, the presence of which does not seem to interfere with the reaction, to yield a completely normal cell wall structure. The vancomycin resistance is represented by seven genes borne on a transposon (Tn1546), allowing them to transfer from bacterium to bacterium (Chapter 10). Three of these genes express enzymes. One of these is a dehydrogenase converting the common cellular metabolite pyruvate to D-lactate. Another enzyme synthesizes D-ala-D-lac, which instead of the normal dipeptide D-ala-D-ala, becomes incorporated at the end of the cross-linking peptide to destroy the binding capacity of the growth-inhibiting vancomycin. The third enzyme, finally, is a peptidase, degrading the normally formed and vancomycin-binding D-ala-D-ala, withdrawing it from competition with the resistance mechanism (Fig. 5.1). As mentioned, the vancomycin resistance is represented by a group of genes borne on a transposon, allowing them to spread from bacterium to bacterium. Where could these genes be imagined to come from? One clue is that lactobacilli, leukonostoc bacteria, and pediococci naturally use a lactate residue instead of a D-alanine at the end of the cross-linking peptide at their transpeptidation reaction. In addition, it has been observed that the vancomycin

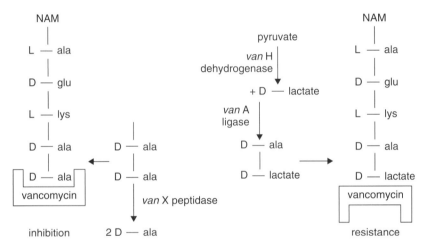

FIGURE 5.1 Transferable vancomycin resistance which is mediated primarily by the three transposon-borne genes *van*H, *van*A, and *van*X. The glycopeptide forming the cross-linking element in the bacterial cell wall (see Chapter 4) is shown schematically with its monosaccharide end NAM (*N*-acetyl muramic acid). The normal peptide is shown to the left with its two D-alanine residues to which vancomycin binds to provide its antibacterial effect by inhibiting the cross-linked cell wall formation. To the right the peptide modified by resistance enzymes is shown. The lactate residue substituting for the normal D-alanine at the end does not bind vankomycin but can participate in a cross-linking reaction. The *van*A gene product is a ligase linking D-alanine to D-lactate for incorporation in the resistance peptide, while *van*H expresses a dehydrogenase turning pyruvate into lactate. The *van*X product is a peptidase supporting the resistance reaction by splitting the D-ala-D-alanine dipeptide to drain it off from the normal vancomycin-susceptible cell wall formation.

resistance gene expressing the D-ala-D-lac synthesizing enzyme has a nucleotide sequence very similar to that of the corresponding gene found in vancomycin-producing bacteria: for example, *Streptomyces toyocaensis*.

There are descriptions of clinical situations where infections with gram-positive pathogens have been completely unresponsive to all available antibacterial agents. The infective agent could, for example, be enterococci resistant to all antibiotics, including vancomycin. Because of case descriptions like that, vancomycin came to be seen as having the almost fateful character as a remedy of last resort. There have been efforts to find small molecules with a selective and catalytically acting activity to degrade the D-ala-D-lac structure of resistance in order to restore the vancomycin-binding ability of the cross-linking peptide. Small molecules with such activity have been identified and shown to lower the vancomycin MIC value eightfold in resistant bacteria. In analogy with a remedy containing clavulanic acid in combination with a betalactam to cope with betalactamases (see Chapter 4), a combination of such small molecules with vancomycin could be able to inhibit resistant cocci.

AVOPARCIN AND CLINICAL RESISTANCE TO GLYCOPEPTIDES

Avoparcin (**5-3**) is a glycopeptide showing structural similarity to vancomycin and teichoplanin. As mentioned in Chapter 2, it was approved in the European Union but not in the United States for use as a growth promoter, particularly in poultry breeding. This practice led to vancomycin resistance appearing in *Enterococcus faecium* of farm animals, spreading into the intestines of urban European adults through the food supply from farms that used avoparcin as a growth promoter. The use of avoparcin for agricultural purposes is now banned, but it was used as a growth promoter for many years. In this context it is ironic that

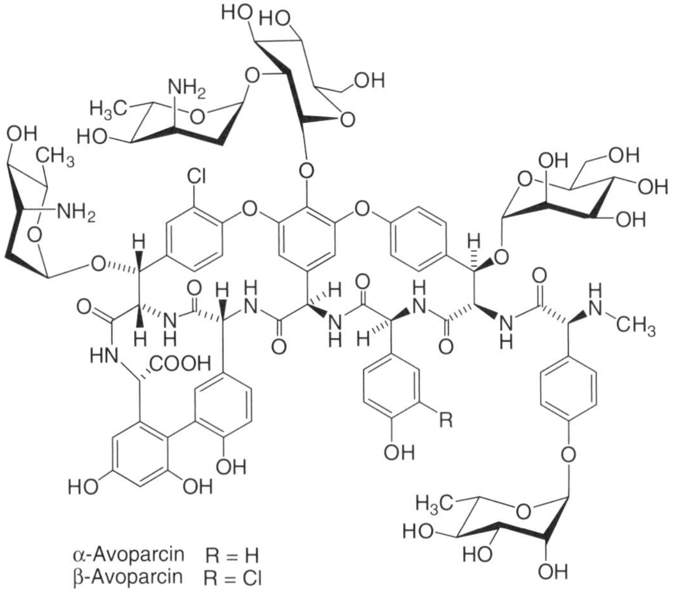

α-Avoparcin R = H
β-Avoparcin R = Cl

Avoparcin

5-3

there were so many very strong European movements against genetically modified crops. The worry extended primarily to the occurrence of resistance genes, usually a betalactamase gene, left in the crop from the genetic construction. In addition to the fact that the betalactamase protein would be destroyed in the food digestion process, it was usually of the simple TEM type, whose occurrence is so frequent anyway that its occurrence in food like this would be of no consequence.

VANCOMYCIN AS AN ANTIBIOTIC OF LAST RESORT

A particularly threatening observation is that vancomycin-resistant enterococci have begun to occur nosocomially at many locations in the world. It has also been shown in laboratory experiments that the seven-membered group of genes mediating vancomycin resistance can be transferred to staphylococci by conjugation. This means that from a microbiological point of view, there is a possibility for the occurrence of vancomycin- and meticillin-resistant *S. aureus* (vancomycin-resistant MRSA). Infections with that type of pathogen would be very difficult to treat—if they could be treated at all. Pathogens of this type have been observed, but luckily they have been rare.)

CHAPTER 6

AMINOGLYCOSIDES

Streptomycin (**6-1**) has been regarded as the second antibiotic discovered (after penicillin) in the history of clinically useful antibacterial agents, and it is an antibiotic in the true sense, isolated originally from the soil organism *Streptomyces griseus*. Streptomycin was discovered at the beginning of the 1940s in the laboratory of Selman Waksman at Rutgers University. Its immediate fame as a remedy depended on its ability to affect *Mycobacterium tuberculosis*. It was the first antibacterial agent that could be used to treat tuberculosis, against which penicillin at that time had no effect. Several antibacterial drugs chemically related to streptomycin have been isolated from other *Streptomyces* species. They are called aminoglycosides after a common feature in their chemical structure. They all work by inhibiting protein synthesis in bacteria. Four aminoglycosides used clinically should be mentioned: tobramycin, gentamicin, amikacin, and netilmicin. The antibacterial action of these four aminoglycosides has a similar mechanism. The molecular mechanisms of resistance to them are also similar. Streptomycin is not used

Antibiotics and Antibiotics Resistance, First Edition. Ola Sköld.
© 2011 John Wiley & Sons, Inc. Published 2011 by John Wiley & Sons, Inc.

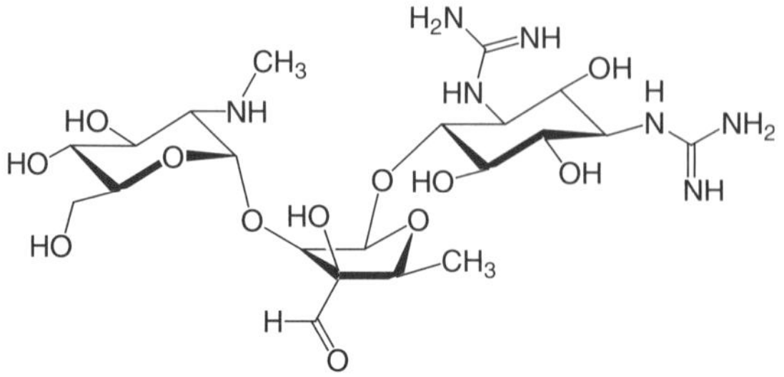

Streptomycin

6-1

nowadays, principally because of its side effects. Most of the streptomycin preparations were taken off pharmacy registration in the 1950s and 1960s, but streptomycin is used here as an example because the microbiological characteristics of amino-glycosides are well described using streptomycin as a model.

THE ANTIBACTERIAL MECHANISM OF STREPTOMYCIN

The chemical structure of streptomycin has three components: streptidine, streptose, and methyl glucoseamine. Streptidine is a cyclohexane derivative with two basic guanidine groups, and streptose is a pentose sugar. The glycosidic bond between the two sugar components streptose and methyl glucosamine has provided the name of this group of antibiotics: the aminoglycosides. The antibacterial effect of streptomycin works by the selective binding of the drug to the smaller part of the bacterial ribosome, inhibiting bacterial protein synthesis. This smaller component of the bacterial ribosome is the 30S particle: S for the Swedberg unit, defining the sedimentation rate of this particle in the gravitational field of an ultracentrifuge. Streptomycin has a broad spectrum of activity, inhibiting both gram-negative and gram-positive bacteria. The selective effect against bacteria is explained by the fact that for structural reasons, aminoglycosides cannot bind to the ribosomes of mammalian cells. Streptomycin cannot be absorbed from the gastrointestinal tract but has to be administered parenterally. This is the rule for all aminoglycosides.

Streptomycin binds very strongly to the bacterial ribosome, one molecule per ribosome inhibiting the peptide synthesis effected by the ribosome. Interaction takes place with the S12 peptide (S for small), one of the 20 peptides, which together with RNA makes up the smaller component, the S30 particle, of the bacterial ribosome. Streptomycin does not bind directly to the S12 peptide, but S12 in some way directs the binding of streptomycin to the ribosome. This is implied further by the fact that a point mutation in S12 leads to streptomycin resistance. If the inhibiting effect of streptomycin on bacterial peptide synthesis is studied in a test tube system, a strange effect can be observed. In a complete system for peptide synthesis in vitro, where the amino acid incorporation is guided by a synthetic polyuridylic acid (polyU) instead of an mRNA transcribed from DNA, an abnormal peptide is formed. PolyU contains one single triplet, UUU, in monotonous repetition, and the peptide formed in such a system is then polyphenylalanine comprised by one repeated amino acid, phenylalanine, corresponding to the triplet UUU of the genetic code. If streptomycin is added to such a system, peptide synthesis is inhibited, as expected, because the drug will bind to the ribosomes present in the in vitro system. If the remaining low peptide synthesis is analyzed closely, it can be seen, however, that the peptide formed contains serine and isoleucine in addition to phenylalanine. This means that streptomycin interferes with the precision of the translation machinery in that the triplet UUU in the presence of streptomycin is also read by the ribosome to direct other amino acids to be incorporated into the peptide formed. This would result in a flow of phenotypic mutations in the growing cell, which would be incompatible with normal cellular functions. On the other hand, it is well known that streptomycin can suppress a number of mutations. This takes place by streptomycin inducing misreading of the mutationally changed triplet as the normal unmutated triplet, resulting finally in the normal peptide. This phenomenon is denoted *phenotypic suppression of mutations*.

BACTERICIDAL EFFECT

Aminoglycosides have a bactericidal effect. This is different from other antibacterial agents affecting bacterial protein synthesis, which are usually bacteriostatic, allowing protein synthesis to proceed in a test tube experiment when the agent has been removed. The bactericidal effect of streptomycin is demonstrated in Figure 6.1, where streptomycin is added to an exponentially growing culture of *E. coli* to the concentration of 30 µg/mL in a test tube. It can be seen that 60 minutes after the addition of streptomycin, only one bacterium in 10,000 of the original population has survived.

An early effect of streptomycin on bacterial cells is to cause leakage of sodium and potassium ions and later also large molecules, which finally kills the cell. There is no immediate explanation of this lethal phenomenon. There are speculations regarding streptomycin-induced misreadings at peptide synthesis with consequent faulty formation of bacterial membrane proteins, resulting in leakage. There is no proof of this, however, and the bactericidal effect of streptomycin is still unexplained.

CLINICAL SIDE EFFECTS

Aminoglycosides have a much feared side effect which was observed very early after the introduction of streptomycin into clinical practice. Aminoglycosides interfere with hearing and with the balance organs of the inner ear. Streptomycin treatment

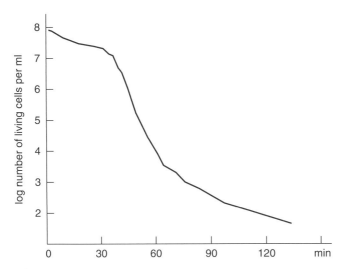

FIGURE 6.1 Bactericidal effect of streptomycin. At time zero, streptomycin was added to a growing liquid culture of *E. coli* and to a concentration of 30 mg/L. The curve shows the number of live bacteria (colony-forming units) on a logarithmic scale.

of tuberculosis in the 1940s and 1950s has left quite a few totally deaf persons into the present time. This severe side effect has been explained by streptomycin binding to and irreversibly damaging cranial nerve eight, which with its branches the cochlearis and vestibularis leads to the inner ear. This is a myth, however, which has been propagated in many, also quite modern, textbooks of microbiology. It is obviously wrong because the eighth cranial nerve is a nerve among others and cannot show a particular specificity for aminoglycosides. Among toxicologists it is well known that aminoglycosides have a toxic effect on the sensory cells of the cochlea and the vestbularis organ. This toxic effect is complicated by the binding of aminoglycosides to the melanin of the cochlea. This explains how the toxic effect can also occur after the drug intake has ceased. Aminoglycoside is set free from melanin after drug treatment has ceased. Interestingly, the ototoxic effect of aminoglycosides has been turned into an advantage by being used skillfully by otolaryngologists to treat the disease of Menière, which runs with disabling fits of rotatory vertigo and also with tinnitus. Initially, systemic treatment with streptomycin was used, resulting in relief from vertigo attacks in many patients—at the price, however, of significant bilateral hearing loss. With another aminoglycoside, gentamicin (**6-2**) (see later in the chapter), whose toxicity seems to be easier to handle, hearing loss could be controlled. Treatment of Menière's disease with gentamicin is performed as a local treatment under an operating microscope by injecting about 10 mg of gentamicin in solution through the eardrum. This dose is repeated for a period of time with close observation of symptoms. Most patients under this treatment become relieved from their disabling vertigo attacks and also to an extent from tinnitus. Gentamicin seems primarily to exert its effect on the sensory hair cells of the vestibular apparatus. In modern clinical practice, aminoglycosides for the treatment of bacterial infections are given in smaller doses than in the early days of streptomycin, and now with close attention to the side effects mentioned, and by continuous assays of drug concentrations in blood serum to guide dosage.

Spectinomycin (**6-3**) is usually regarded as a member of the aminoglycoside group of antibiotics, despite the fact that it does

Gentamicin C_1 R = R′ = CH_3

Gentamicin C_2 R = CH_3 R′ = H

Gentamicin C_{1a} R = R′ = H

Gentamicin

6-2

Spectinomycin

6-3

not contain any amino sugar residue. Its structure is that of an aminocyclitol. Unlike the other aminoglycoside antibiotics mentioned it acts bacteriostatically rather than bactericidally. Its effects on the protein synthesis are also different from those of the other aminoglycosides. It does not, for example, induce misreadings as does streptomycin, which was mentioned earlier in the chapter. As *Neisseria gonorrhoeae* acquired betalactamase to emerge as a pathogen resistant to betalactams, spectinomycin found a very useful clinical application in the treatment of the sexually transmitted disease gonorrhea.

BACTERIAL RESISTANCE TO AMINOGLYCOSIDES

The simplest form of bacterial resistance to streptomycin is effected by point mutations in the S12 peptide of the smaller component of the bacterial ribosome, the S30 particle, to which streptomycin binds. This type of resistance is easy to find experimentally by growing *E. coli* bacteria spread out on an agar plate containing a low concentration of streptomycin. Spontaneous mutants to resistance will then be observed at a low frequency. Upon closer analysis these mutations are found to be expressed as amino acid changes located in the S12 peptide and diminishing the binding of streptomycin to the ribosome, resulting in a lower inhibition effect. Several amino acid changes in S12 are known to result in streptomycin resistance. Some mutations not only result in resistance but strangely enough also in streptomycin

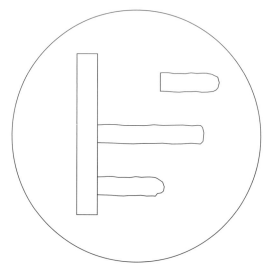

FIGURE 6.2 Susceptibility and resistance to, and dependence on, strep-tomycin. *E. coli* was grown on an agar plate with a filter paper strip impregnated with streptomycin, causing a concentration gradient in the agar medium. The upper growth shows susceptibility; the middle, resistance; and the lowest, dependence.

dependence. This is illustrated in Figure 6.2, where the bacterial streak at the bottom shows diminishing growth with the diminishing concentration of streptomycin in the gradient from a filter paper strip impregnated with streptomycin. This phenomenon could be understood by the important function of the ribosome in the precise decoding of the mRNA nucleotide sequence. The mutation to dependence could be thought of as increasing the fidelity requirement at codon recognition to such an extent that it is inhibited and for translation to proceed needs that earlier mentioned misreading induced by streptomycin.

HORIZONTAL SPREAD OF AMINOGLYCOSIDE RESISTANCE

High resistance to streptomycin and other aminoglycosides in clinical contexts is usually mediated by horizontally transferred genes expressing drug-inactivating enzymes in pathogenic bacteria. These inactivating reactions are of three types: phosphorylation, adenylylation, and acetylation, by which the aminoglycoside is modified to make it unable to bind to the bacterial ribosome. To continue with streptomycin as an aminoglycoside example, there are the resistance-mediating enzymes that O-phosphorylate and O-adenylylate streptomycin. The target is the hydroxyl group on the third carbon atom of the aminoglucose component of the streptomycin molecule (see formula **6-1** and Fig. 6.3), and with another specificity, the hydroxyl group of the sixth carbon atom in the cyclohexane component. At phosphorylation the phosphate source is ATP, which also delivers the adenyl group at adenylylation, with inorganic pyrophosphate as a rest product.

No acetylating enzyme with streptomycin as a substrate has been observed, but with the aminoglycoside gentamicin (see **6-2**), acetylating enzymes inactivating the drug have been seen and with an amino group as a target. The acetyl source is acetyl coenzyme A. The aminocyclitol mentioned, spectinomycin, which is included among the aminoglycosides, is inactivated by an O-adenylylation enzyme. The phosphorylating, adenylylating, and acetylating enzymes form groups with several interrelated members, with varying substrate specificities for different aminoglycosides. An extensive cross resistance follows from these conditions. In this context a very interesting observation may be made. Clinical isolates of *E. coli* were shown to carry aminoglycoside acetylating enzymes, the substrate specificity of which was seen to have changed mutationally to include a completely unrelated substrate, ciprofloxacin, which is a quinolone (see Chapter 8).These isolates thus showed quinolone resistance. The ciprofloxacin was observed to be N-acetylated at its piperazinyl substituent (see **8-2**). The quinolones, including ciprofloxacin, are synthetic, so bacteria could not have encountered compounds like that before they were introduced clinically as antibacterials

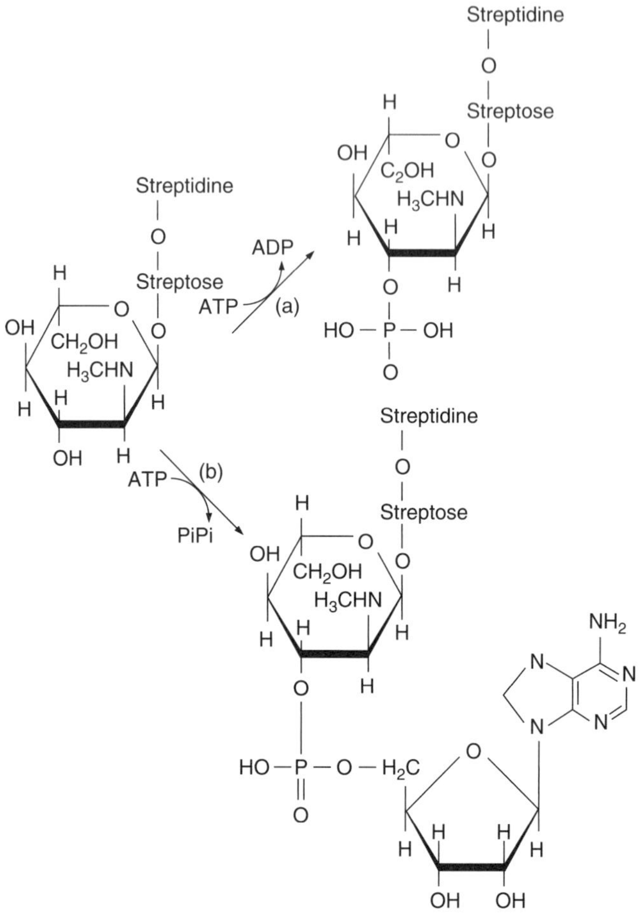

FIGURE 6.3 Inactivation of streptomycin by transferable resistance enzymes: (a) phosphorylation; (b) adenylylation.

in the 1960s. This is at variance with the idea that antibiotic-inactivating enzymes have evolved during a very long time in bacteria exposed to naturally occurring antibiotics, and that these enzymes probably originated in the antibiotic-producing organisms. The gene responsible for this acetylation phenomenon is a variant of one that encodes an enzyme with a chemically different but clinically related substrate that is an antibiotic of another class. This is thus the evolution of a gene with a new function, again illustrating the amazing ability of bacteria to adapt to our use of antibacterial remedies.

The genes for aminoglycoside-inactivating enzymes spread horizontally by transposons and plasmids (see Chapter 10), and their origins can then be questioned. It has been shown that the resistance mechanisms mentioned can also be found in aminoglycoside-producing soil organisms such as *S. griseus*. They can be regarded there as suicide protection (i.e., an organism killing itself with its own antibiotic products).

CONCLUSION

The clinical use of aminoglycosides has to be supervised carefully because of their serious side effects, which limit their present distribution. They are also very interesting from a microbiological point of view. Studies of their mechanisms of action have to a large extent contributed to an understanding of ribosomal function at bacterial peptide synthesis. That aminoglycoside resistance mechanisms, similar to those found in pathogenic bacteria, can also be found in soil organisms is probably a key to the origin of most enzymes that mediate resistance to antibiotics.

CHAPTER 7

OTHER ANTIBIOTICS INTERFERING WITH BACTERIAL PROTEIN SYNTHESIS

Streptomycin and other aminoglycosides were the first antibiotics used clinically to act selectively on bacterial protein synthesis. Further antibacterial agents inhibiting bacterial peptide synthesis are described in this chapter: among them the frequently used tetracyclines and the macrolides, also chloramphenicol, feared for its side effects, and the rarely used fusidic acid. Finally, the last new, selectively acting antibacterial agent, linezolid, is described, together with its effect on bacterial protein synthesis by means of an earlier unknown mechanism.

CHLORAMPHENICOL

Chloramphenicol (**7-1**) is an antibiotic in the true sense. It was isolated from *Streptomyces venezuelae* in 1947 and was introduced in clinical medicine in the 1950s. Its molecular structure is rather simple. Chloramphenicol is now produced industrially by chemical synthesis. The effect of chloramphenicol, which

Antibiotics and Antibiotics Resistance, First Edition. Ola Sköld.
© 2011 John Wiley & Sons, Inc. Published 2011 by John Wiley & Sons, Inc.

Chloramphenicol

7-1

acts by inhibiting bacterial protein synthesis, is reversible and thus bacteriostatic. Experiments with radioactively labeled chloramphenicol have shown its exclusive binding to the larger, 50S subunit of the bacterial ribosome (70S), one molecule per 50S particle. It does not bind at all to mammalian 80S ribosomes, which explaines its selective action on bacteria. As noted earlier, the Swedberg unit defines the movement of the particle in the gravitational field of an ultracentrifuge. Simple experiments explain the reversible bacteriostatic effect of chloramphenicol, in that the drug can easily be removed from a bacterial culture, by centrifugation or filtration, allowing the bacterial ribosomes to resume their normal function. This has been an important tool in earlier investigations of the interplay between protein synthesis and the formation of other macromolecules in the bacterial cell, by allowing the temporary inhibition of protein synthesis. Specifically, chloramphenicol binds to several peptides of the 50S particle, including L15, L18, and L27 (L for large, the larger subunit of the 70S bacterial ribosome). Chloramphenicol also seems to bind to a specific area, the V-domain, of the 23S rRNA, which together with 55 peptides is a main component of the complete ribosome and which effects the peptide bond formation (i.e., the main reaction of peptide formation). These observations do not, however, allow a complete understanding of protein synthesis inhibition by chloramphenicol, the details of which remain to be explained.

Chloramphenicol was one of the first antibiotics with a broad spectrum: that is, with an effect against both gram-positive and gram-negative bacteria, inhibiting most pathogenic bacteria. Chloramphenicol also has the ability to pass through the blood–brain barrier. In the liquor cerebrospinalis it reaches concentrations that are 30 to 50% of those in the blood serum, which means that this drug can be used efficiently for the treatment of meningitis.

Clinical Side Effects

Chloramphenicol ought to be a much appreciated antibiotic for the systemic treatment of bacterial infections—but it is not. It is used principally for external purposes, as in skin ointments and eyedrops. This is because of a feared side effect, blood dyscrasias, which occur in two forms, one dose related and reversible, the other dose independent, appearing late in the treatment and mediating an irreversible and fatal aplastic anemia. The latter side effect has a low incidence, about one in 200,000 cases treated, but still has led to a very limited use of this drug in clinical praxis. The precise etiology of this side effect is not known. It has been speculated that the known inhibition of mitocondrial protein synthesis in mammalian cells by chloramphenicol could play a role, but this is not consistent with the very low incidence of this side effect. In later years the sensitivity to chloramphenicol and the appearance of aplastic anemia have been shown to have a hereditary component, which has not been defined further. In severe infectious diseases such as meningitis and typhoid fever, when the risk of the disease and the risk of side effects are in the balance, chloramphenicol is a very valuable antibacterial agent.

Bacterial Resistance to Chloramphenicol

Resistance to chloramphenicol occurs in two forms. One is easily observed in the laboratory by growing experimental bacteria at incrementally increasing concentrations of chloramphenicol. This resistance is explained by a decreased permeability occurring in steps and induced by spontaneous mutations. The clinically most important form of resistance is of another type, however, mediated by an enzymatic inactivation of chloramphenicol by the acetylation of its two hydroxyl groups (see **7-1**). This acetylation is effected by foreign genes expressing chloramphenicol acetyl transferases by transferring an acetyl group from acetyl coenzymeA to the outer of the two hydroxyl groups in the chloramphenicol molecule. This acetyl group then migrates nonenzymically to the inner hydroxyl group. The outer hydroxyl group is again acetylated by an acetyl transferase to give a final product, diacetyl chloramphenicol. The two acetyl groups prevent the binding of chloramphenicol to the bacterial ribosome, invalidating its antibacterial effect.

Chloramphenicol acetylating enzymes can be observed in both gram-negative and gram-positive bacteria, and their corresponding genes are located chromosomally or borne on plasmids. In the latter case they are likely to be transferable horizontally (see Chapter 10). One chloramphenicol acetyl transferase common among gram-negative enterobacteria is borne on a transposon, Tn9. The chloramphenicol acetyl transferases transferring between pathogens and mediating clinical resistance probably have their origins among chloramphenicol-producing soil organisms, where they protect the producing organism against its own product. Resistance against chloramphenicol was among the first horizontally transferred resistance properties discovered in a clinical context, observed in the early 1950s in Japan during epidemics of bacterial dysentery. It could be seen that patients excreting antibiotic-susceptible *Shigella* bacteria at the beginning of the infection, later and after antibiotic treatment excreted multiply-resistant bacteria carrying resistance to chloramphenicol, streptomycin, tetracycline, and sulfonamides, despite the fact that they had been treated with only one of these agents. In further observations, patients were seen to excrete both susceptible and multiresistant *Shigella* bacteria of the same bacterial serotype. All these observations were interpreted by two Japanese microbiologists, Tomoichiro Akiba and Kunitaro Ochiai, to mean that genes mediating resistance to all four antibiotics were located on a transferable plasmid with the ability to wander from bacterium to bacterium via conjugation (more about this in Chapter 10).

TETRACYCLINES

There is another group of antibiotics that interfere with bacterial protein synthesis and with their origin in soil bacteria: tetracyclines (**7-2**), produced in many *Streptomyces* species. The name hints at their chemical structure, with a four-membered ring structure carrying several functional groups, varying in microbiological origin—hence the plural form. The structure shown represents the tetracycline originally isolated from *Streptomyces viridifaciens*; oxytetracycline, isolated from *S. rimosus*, has a hydroxyl group instead of hydrogen at the bottom of the third ring of the tetracycline. Doxycycline lacks two hydroxyl groups: one in each of the second and third rings. Several tetracyclines with further variations in the functional groups are known, but since the antibacterial spectrum and mechanism of action are very similar among them, and since bacteria show cross resistance against them, from a microbiological point of view they could be regarded as identical. Tetracyclines are effective against many different pathogens and are regarded as

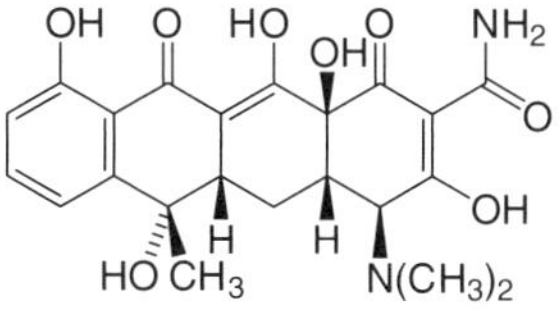

Tetracycline

7-2

broad-spectrum antibiotics that also have an effect against rickettsiae, mycoplasma, and certain protozoa (e.g., malaria). The very good ability of tetracyclines to heal acne seems to depend not only on an antibacterial effect against *Propionibacterium acnes* but also on an unspecific anti-inflammatory effect.

Mechanism of Action

Tetracyclines act bacteriostatically by reversibly inhibiting the bacterial peptide synthesis. They bind to to the 70S ribosome and inhibit the binding of the amino acid carrying tRNA molecule to the ribosome. A site with a high affinity for tetracycline has been identified on the 30S subunit of the 70S ribosome. Tetracyclines also bind to and inhibit the function of eucaryotic 80S ribosomes, but to a much more limited extent, which explains the selectivity. Bacteria also have the capability of concentrating tetracyclines into their cells by cell pump mechanisms. The exact mechanism of interaction between tetracyclines and bacterial ribosomes to inhibit bacterial peptide synthesis is not known. It could be mentioned that tetracyclines do not interfere with the binding of chloramphenicol to bacterial ribosomes.

Four tetracycline derivatives are in most common use in clinical praxis: tetracycline, oxytetracycline, doxycycline, and lymecycline. As mentioned, they are identical in antibacterial action but differ in pharmacokinetic behavior. Lumecycline, for example, is a tetracycline ligated to the amino acid lysine, which facilitates the absorbtion and is rapidly hydrolyzed off during passage through the gut wall to release tetracycline. Tigecycline is another derivative carrying a glycine substitution. It is to some extent active against pathogens resistant to other tetracyclines. It is used as a remedy against methicillin-resistant staphylococci (MRSA). Tigecycline marketed under the brand name Tygacil is only available for parenteral administration.

Clinical Side Effects

Tetracyclines have the chemical property of forming insoluble chelate compounds with divalent cations: for example, calcium (Ca^{2+}) and iron (Fe^{2+}). When tetracycline ingestion takes place in combination with iron given for the treatment of anemia or together with milk (Ca^{2+}), uptake is interfered with. This chemical property of the tetracyclines also gives them a high affinity for growing bone tissue and for growing teeth. This can result in miscoloring of teeth and interfere with tooth growth as a consequence. Tetracyclines should not be prescribed to children under the age of 8 or to pregnant women.

Bacterial Resistance to Tetracyclines

Tetracyclines have been used very widely in both humans and animals because of their efficient antibacterial effect, their broad spectrum of effectiveness, their mild and managable side effects, and their low cost. Tetracyclines have also been used in sub-therapeutic doses added to fodder to promote growth in animal breeding. The microbial world has responded to this large and wide distribution of tetracyclines by developing resistance, which is now notably limiting their clinical efficiency. Many pathogenic and commensal bacteria are now tetracycline resistant through harboring *tet* resistance genes, of which now more than 30 different types have been identified and characterized. They have been shown to have their origin in tetracycline-producing *Streptomyces* species, where they can be regarded as protection against the antibiotics they produce themselves. The very fast spread of the *tet* genes into and between pathogenic bacteria is a reflection of the efficiency of those genetic mechanisms that allow the horizontal spread of genes among bacteria. This is described in more detail in Chapter 10. The *tet* genes express two types of tetracycline resistance proteins, in turn mediating two types of resistance. One type, the efflux proteins, about 46 kDa in size, are incorporated into the cytoplasmic membrane of the bacterial cell and work by pumping out tetracyclines of the cell under the consumption of energy, thus protecting the ribosomes from inhibiting concentrations of the drug. The other type of protein occurs in cytoplasma and protects the bacterial ribosomes by binding to them and changing their conformation to disallow tetracycline binding while allowing a concomitant normal protein synthesis to proceed. The affinity of these resistance proteins for bacterial ribosomes is explained partially by their structural analogy with the elongation factors of the protein-synthesizing machinery, which also bind to the ribosomes. The effect of these ribosome-binding resistance proteins can also be demonstrated in a test tube system, which cannot be done with the efflux proteins, which require cellular integrity and intact bacterial membranes. It should be mentioned here that this tetracycline resistance mechanism with ribosome-protecting proteins has not been found in gram-negative enterobacteria, probably because this mechanism would effect only a low resistance in these enterobacteria.

The general increase and spread of tetracycline resistance, assisted by transferable plasmids, transposons, and integrons (see Chapter 10), has been dramatic. It has drastically curbed the usability of these efficient and inexpensive broad-spectrum antibiotics. Recently, promising attempts have been made to modify the tetracycline molecule chemically to decrease its affinity for the resistance proteins. The best derivative so far in these modifying attempts has been a pentacycline, a chemical structure of five rings. Also tigecycline, a glycylcycline, a glycine derivative, has been developed as a clinical agent to circumvent the tetracycline resistance mechanisms. With its large hydrophobic group, glycylcycline displays activity against strains expressing genes for tetracycline resistance, including those that encode ribosomal protection and efflux mechanisms.This could be due to the failure of efflux proteins to recognize glycylcycline or to the inability of these proteins to translocate glycylcycline across the cytoplasmic membrane even though these proteins may recognize and bind the new analog. The result of either mechanism would be failure to remove glycylcycline from the bacterial cytoplasm so that inhibitor concentrations necessary to prevent protein synthesis would be maintained. Glycylcycline competes with tetracyline for ribosomal binding but has a higher binding affinity than that of earlier tetracyclines. This is probably why ribosomal protection proteins are unable to confer resistance to glycylcycline.

ERYTHROMYCIN AND RELATED ANTIBIOTICS

Macrolides, lincosamides, and streptogramins are three groups of antibiotics that are classified together despite the fact that they are structurally very different but have similar mechanisms of action and meet with the same type of resistance. Together they are termed the MLS group.

Macrolides

Erythromycin (**7-3**) serves as a good example of the macrolide group. It was discovered in 1952 as an antibiotic produced by *Streptomyces erythreus*. Its chemical structure is rather complex, and it is characterized by a large lactone ring to which two sugar molecules, one of which is an amino sugar, are bound by glycoside bonds. Erythromycin selectively inhibits bacterial growth by binding to bacterial ribosomes, where it reversibly inhibits protein synthesis. The selective action of erythromycin is explained by its inability to bind to and to inhibit the function of mammalian ribosomes. Its reversible action on bacterial ribosomes means that its antimicrobial effect is bacteriostatic. Closer

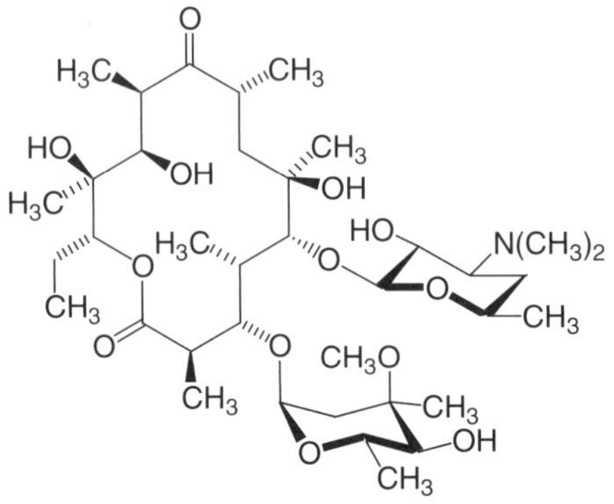

Erythromycin

7-3

studies have shown that erythromycin binds to the 50S particle of the bacterial ribosome, one molecule per 50S particle, and that the 23S RNA, the nucleus of the 50S particle, is involved in the binding. It ought to be mentioned that erythromycin and chloramphenicol do not compete in ribosome binding. Erythromycin inhibits ribosomal peptide synthesis by interfering with the binding of aminoacyl-tRNA to the ribosome and thus inhibiting the peptide elongation.

Erythromycin has a good effect against a rather broad spectrum of gram-positive pathogenic bacteria and also against a few gram-negative bacteria. It is used against respiratory infections and particularly to substitute for penicillin for the treatment of patients allergic to this drug. It is also a standard component of the combination treatment of peptic ulcer caused by *Helicobacter pylori*.

Resistance to Erythromycin

The methylation of a specific adenine in the nucleotide sequence of the 23S RNA of the bacterial ribosome is associated with resistance to erythromycin. This adenine residue has been identified as A-2058 in the 23S-RNA nucleotide sequence. The A-2058 is normally not methylated, but at erythromycin resistance it is methylated or dimethylated at the amino group of its seventh carbon atom. This methylation seems to change the tertiary structure of that 23S RNA domain effecting the peptide synthesis, such that erythromycin binding and peptide synthesis inhibition is abolished. This methylation is enzymatic and is effected by a group of N-methyl transferases that have the ability to transfer a methyl group to adenine, in this case with S-adenosylmethionine as a donor. In erythromycin-resistant pathogens such as staphylococci and streptococci, these enzymes are expressed from plasmid-borne *erm* genes, many of which are known and characterized. Some of these have the ability to transfer two methyl groups, whereas others transfer only one. Dimethylases mediate a higher degree of resistance and to a wider variety of macrolides than those that transfer only one.

Clinical Use of Macrolides

Five different macrolides are used most frequently in clinical contexts: erythromycin, roxithromycin, klarithromycin, azithromycin, and telithromycin. Of these, four are semisynthetic derivatives of erythromycin with microbiological properties very similar to those of erythromycin. The mechanism of antibacterial action is the same for all five and the bacterial mechanism of resistance is common. This means that there is cross resistance between members of the group.

Lincosamides

Lincomycin (**7-4**) was discovered in the 1960s and shown to be an antibiotic product of *Streptomyces lincolnensis*. It has a rather simple chemical structure with an amino sugar in an amide bond to a heterocyclic, five-membered, nitrogen-containing ring. Its

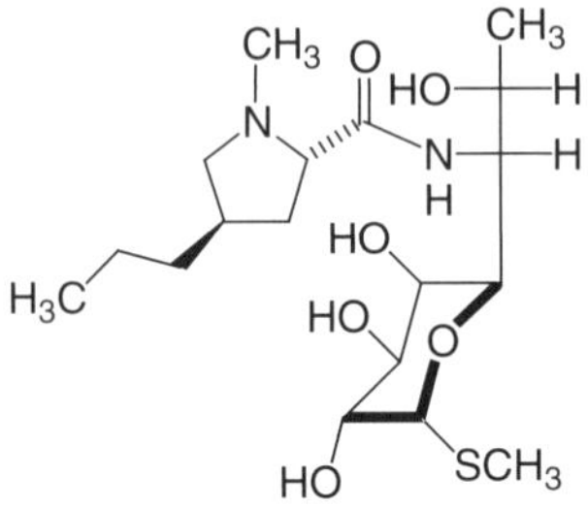

Lincomycin

7-4

structure is thus very different from that of macrolides, but its antibacterial mechanism is very similar, by binding to the 50S particle of the bacterial ribosome. Lincomycin acts selectively on bacteria by not binding to the ribosomes of mammalian cells. Resistance to lincomycin is mediated by N-dimethylation of A-2058 as with macrolides, indicating a similar type of ribosome binding and also cross resistance with macrolides.

A close analog to linkomycin, clindamycin, which has similar antimicrobial properties, has found clinical use. It shows an effect against anaerobic pathogens such as *Bacteroides*. This property is linked to a much feared side effect. Clindamycin in the anaerobic environment of the human gut will select for the pathogenic *Bacterium difficile*, which is endogenously resistant to clindamycin. This bacterium produces toxins that damage the intestinal wall of the colon, resulting in a potentially lethal condition of pseudomembraneous colitis. As mentioned in Chapter 5, vancomycin can then be a lifesaving remedy.

Streptogramins

Further antibiotics of the MLS group are streptogramins. They have their origin in soil bacteria such as *Streptomyces graminofaciens*. The streptogramins vary among themselves and with their origins in different *Streptomyces* species, but pairwise they have a similar structure, a similar mechanism of action, and similar antibacterial spectra. They occur in pairs of two forms, A and B, which have very different structures, in the various streptogramin-producing *Streptomyces* species. The two forms act in synergy for antibacterial action by binding to the ribosomal 50S particles to cause an irreversible inhibition of bacterial peptide synthesis. The irreversibility of protein synthesis inhibition means that streptogramins have a bactericidal effect. Despite the very large structural differences among streptogramins, lincosamides, and macrolides, they bind similarly to the bacterial ribosome to inhibit bacterial peptide synthesis. The antibacterial similarity is also demonstrated by the fact that the dimethylation of adenine-2058 in the ribosomal 23S RNA mediates resistance against all three antibiotic groups.

The streptogramins have been known for several decades, but came into clinical use only in recent years, primarily because the worsening resistance situation has forced clinicians to use antibiotics regarded as being difficult to handle. One streptogramin preparation, Synercid, containing the A form dalfopristine and the B form kinopristine in the proportion 70 : 30, has been used against vancomycin-resistant staphylococci and streptococci. This use has been regarded as clinically important and necessary despite such side effects as arthritis and general muscle pain. One form of streptogramin B, virginiamycin, has long been used in the United States to promote growth in husbandry animals. This has given rise to Synercid-resistant gram-positive pathogens with the potential to spread to human infections. This is an example of the risk of spreading antibiotic resistance from husbandry animals to human beings by the uncontrolled use of antibiotics. The common resistance mechanism of RNA methylation in macrolides, lincosamides, and streptogramins means that there is cross resistance among the members of the MLS group.

FUSIDIC ACID

From a structural point of view, fusidic acid (**7-5**) is unique among antibiotics. It was originally isolated from the mold *Fusidium coccineum* in 1962 by a group of Danish researchers in Copenhagen. It is thus an antibiotic in the true sense of the word. The name *fusidic acid* was coined by the discoverers. *F. coccineum* lives on the leaves of plants. Fusidic acid is structurally a steroid but has no pharmacological effect. It has a narrow spectrum of antibacterial effect directed primarily toward *Staphylococcus aureus* but also against coagulase-negative staphylococci, corynebacteria, and clostridia. Its clinical use is mainly as a *Staphylococcus* antibiotic. Fusidic acid has a good penetrating ability, which makes it useful at staphylococcal infections in less well vascularized tissues such as bone in osteomyelitis.

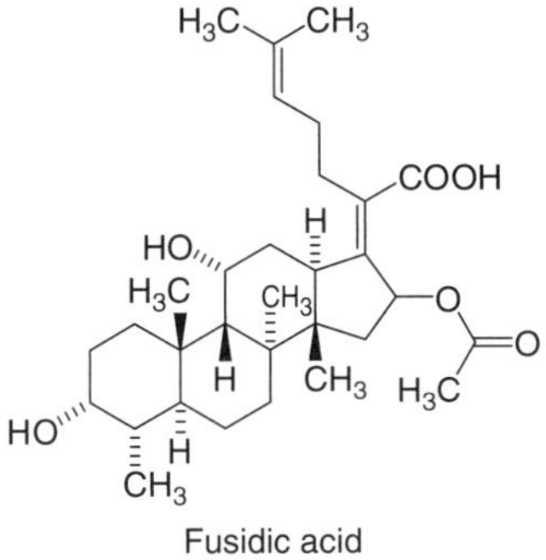

Fusidic acid

7-5

Fusidic acid works by interfering with bacterial protein synthesis, and more specifically by binding to and inhibiting the function of the peptide elongation factor EF-G. A corresponding inhibition can be observed in test tube experiments with components from mammalian cells. Still, fusidic acid has a selective action against bacteria, probably because it cannot reach inhibitory concentration in mammalian cells, which show a low permeability for the drug. Resistance against fusidic acid has been observed and is effected by spontaneous mutations, diminishing the affinity of elongation factor EF-G for the drug. Also, plasmid-borne resistance to fusidic acid has been suggested to occur and then mediated by plasmid-borne genes for the synthesis of cell wall components, diminishing the cellular uptake of fusidic acid. Observations of such phenomena and their intrepretations are still preliminary, however, and have not been verified.

LINEZOLID

Oxazolidinones comprise a group of synthetic substances which have been known for 30 years for their antibacterial activity. They are mentioned in an American patent from 1978. Their antibacterial effect was originally discovered in screening experiments of a large number of chemical compounds. Two of these compounds, linezolid (**7-6**) and eperezolid (**7-7**), have found use as antibacterial agents. The heterocyclic, nitrogen-containing, five-membered ring is oxazolidinon, which has given its name to the entire group of substances. Linezolid is registered as an antibacterial drug under the name Zyvox. Linezolid is most effective against gram-positive cocci and is useful in the treatment of methicillin-resistant staphylococci (MRSA).

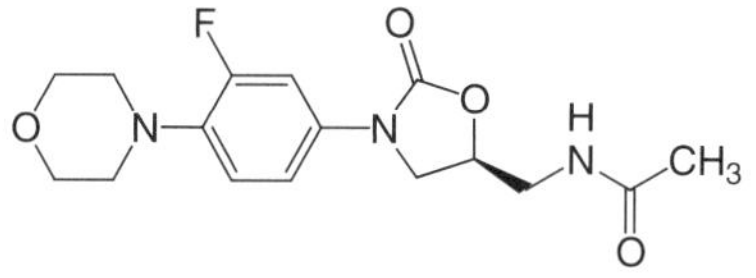

Linezolid

7-6

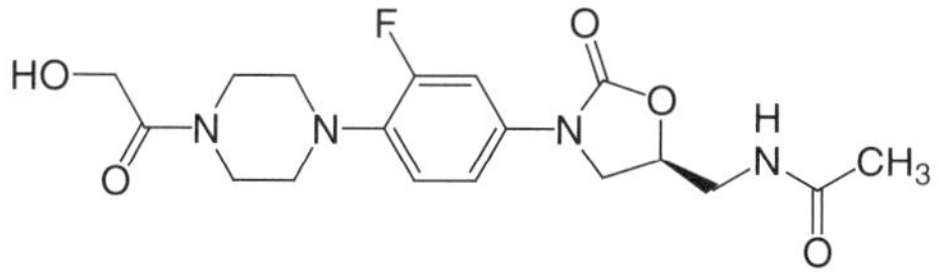

Eperezolid

7-7

As mentioned earlier, most antibacterial agents can be looked at as members of large groups or families within which cross resistance is common. This is because the group members have the same basic mechanism of action (see Chapter 11). From a resistance point of view it is therefore important to find antibacterial agents with a new mechanism of action—so new and different that the world of pathogenic bacteria has not seen it before. In this sense, linezolid is a truly new antibacterial drug. A truly new antibacterial agent such as linezolid has not been added to the antibiotic arsenal since the introduction of trimethoprim at the end of the 1960s. Linezolid works by selectively inhibiting bacterial protein synthesis. This is also the mechanism of action of many other antibacterials, such as tetracyclines, aminoglycosides, and chloramphenicol, but linezolid and other oxazolidinones have a different and for antibacterial agents a new mode of inhibition, in that they inhibit initiation of the bacterial peptide synthesis. This process of peptide formation requires the cooperation of several large structures and molecules, such as ribosomes, on the surface of which peptide bonds are formed, and mRNA mediating and controlling the amino acid sequence according to the gene representing the particular protein being formed. For the peptide synthesis to get started, a set of specific components is also needed. Among them is a particular tRNA molecule, formylmethionyl-tRNA, carrying the initiating amino acid, methionine, to the peptide start point on the ribosome. Bacterial ribosomes are built of large RNA molecules and about 100 peptides. Their complete structure and function are not known precisely, despite decades of intensive research. The precise mechanism of action for linezolid is not known either. Detailed experiments seem to show that the agent binds to the ribosome to change the binding locus of the initiation tRNA and thus derail the initiation of peptide synthesis. The new mechanism of action and the fact that linezolid is a synthetic agent ought to mean that resistance to it should at least be delayed. Spontaneous mutants have been isolated, however, showing a changed ribosome structure, mediating a lowered binding of linezolid, resulting in resistance. Also, clinical isolates of several gram-positive cocci, among them *Staphylococcus aureus*, have shown resistance. This is in parallel to what has been observed for other synthetic antibacterial agents, such as quinolones (i.e. mutationally changed target structures; see Chapter 8).

CONCLUSION

The antibacterial agents described in this chapter have only one thing in common: They all selectively inhibit bacterial protein synthesis. Otherwise, they are very different in chemical structure, mechanisms of action, and in many cases also in clinical use. These substances, possibly with the exception of linezolid, could be viewed as agents that evolution has brought forth as a means of competition among soil bacteria, which we have discovered, isolated, and put to use in fighting bacterial disease. Resistance development tells us, however, that we only seem to have them on loan.

CHAPTER 8

QUINOLONES

Nalidixic acid (**8-1**) is the original substance of the group of synthetic antibacterial agents called quinolones. It was discovered in a synthesis program originally based on observation of the antibacterial properties of an oxoquinoline, found as a by-product of the industrial synthesis of the malaria drug chloroquine. This observation and a follow-up screening program occurred at the beginning of the 1960s and has, starting with nalidixic acid, produced a number of synthetic derivatives which have become one of the most important groups of remedies in antibacterial

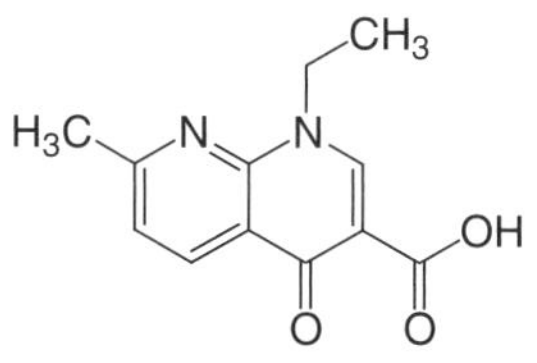

Nalidixic acid

8-1

Antibiotics and Antibiotics Resistance, First Edition. Ola Sköld.
© 2011 John Wiley & Sons, Inc. Published 2011 by John Wiley & Sons, Inc.

therapy. They are distributed as inexpensive and efficient antibacterial agents, particularly against urinary tract infections
caused by gram-negative enterobacteria.

THE EFFECT OF QUINOLONES ON BACTERIA

Quinolones have a selective and bactericidal effect by interfering
with bacterial DNA replication. However, they do not interfere
with the synthesis of DNA but with those changes in conformation that the DNA molecule has to go through at replication
and cell division. The molecular length of bacterial DNA is about
1300 μm, while the typical bacterial cell has a diameter of about
1 μm. To become accommodated in the daughter cells, after
replication the two DNA copies have to adapt to a more compact
structure by supercoiling to a knotlike form (Fig. 8.1). There is
a mundane comparison to explain this: The long DNA chain is
compared with a telephone cord that gets twinned and finally
overtwinned by many rotations of the receiver when answering
and hanging up. In the end the telephoning person has to sit
with her head very close to the phone. The overtwinning of
DNA is negative; that is, it runs in the direction opposite to the
spiral structure of the DNA and is effected enzymically by DNA
gyrase, which works by cutting both DNA strands to let another
part of the circular double-stranded molecule pass through the
break, which is then sealed by another enzymic gyrase function
(Fig. 8.1). The gyrase enzyme has four pairwise identical subunits: two A subunits (97 kDa) and two B subunits (90 kDa).
During the course of the enzymic reaction the two DNA strands
are cut and become covalently bound to the two A subunits. This
prohibits rotation of the double strand. The quinolones work by
binding to the enzyme–DNA complex in this condition, thus
inhibiting religation of the cut DNA strands. The overtwinning
reaction, which is very important for replication of the bacterial

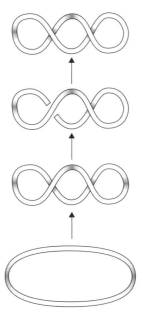

FIGURE 8.1   Enzymic effect of bacterial DNA gyrase. The gyrase enzyme binds to a circular DNA molecule to induce formation of the stylized structure second from the bottom of the figure. The enzyme then cuts both DNA strands to create a gap through which the other DNA segment can pass (third from the bottom), to form a first structural step (fourth from the bottom), toward supercoiling.

cell, is then irreversibly stopped halfway, leading to cell death, because the stalled step in the final formation of cellular DNA will eventually be recognized by the cellular enzymes for DNA error correction leading to DNA degradation. Quinolones thus have a bactericidal effect. The corresponding enzymes with gyrase function in human mammalian cells are structurally so different that they are not recognized by the quinolones, which are then selective in their action on bacteria.

There are further enzymes of the bacterial cell modifying DNA structure: for example, releasing overtwinning to allow transcription and DNA replication, commonly called topoisomerases. One of these, topoisomerase IV, releasing the chain structure (decatenation) of newly replicated DNA, is inhibited by quinolones, but to a lesser extent. The most important bacterial target for quinolones is the DNA gyrase.

CLINICAL USE OF QUINOLONES

As mentioned earlier, nalidixic acid was the first quinolone used clinically. From a microbiological point of view, it was then a new antibacterial agent against which the microbial world had not selected resistance. Compare the argument regarding antibiotic families in Chapter 11. Also, the quinolones are synthetic agents that the microbial world could not be expected to have come across earlier in its history. Nalidixic acid had to be given in very large doses, however, with side effects occurring. The antibacterial effect was very much enhanced by the introduction of 6-fluoro and 5-piperidine groups in the molecule, to allow lower doses for the clinical effect. This important breakthrough for the antibacterial use of quinolones was made by Japanese chemists in the mid-1970s, and allowed the introduction of that larger group of quinolones, today being very important in the treatment of bacterial infections. As examples of these fluoroquinolones, ciprofloxacin (**8-2**), norfloxacin (**8-3**), ofloxacin (**8-4**), levofloxacin (**8-5**), and moxifloxacin (**8-6**) could be mentioned. They all have the mechanism of action described earlier and have similar antibacterial spectra. The quinolones mentioned are

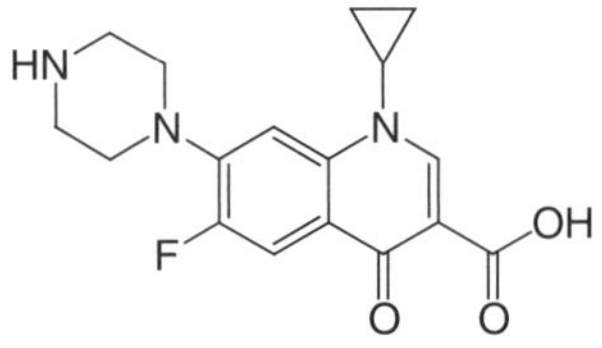

Ciprofloxacin

8-2

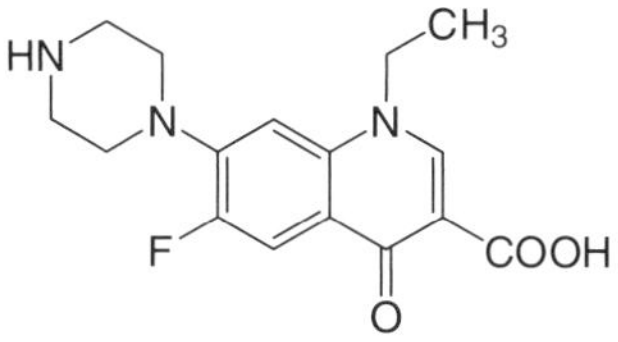

Norfloxacin

8-3

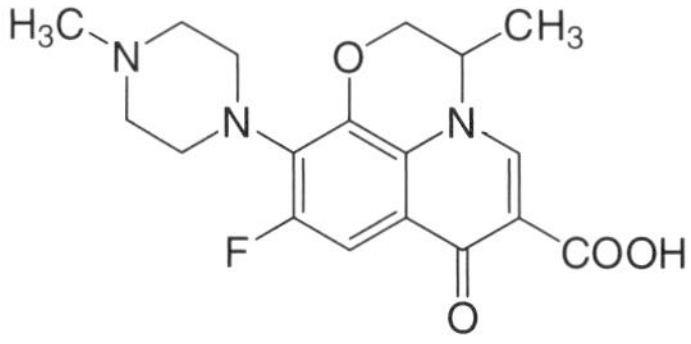

Ofloxacin

8-4

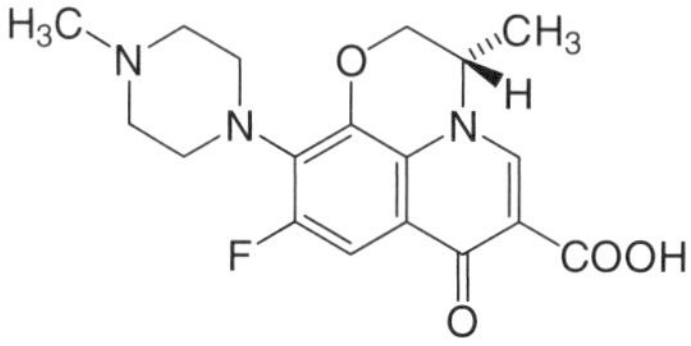

Levofloxacin

8-5

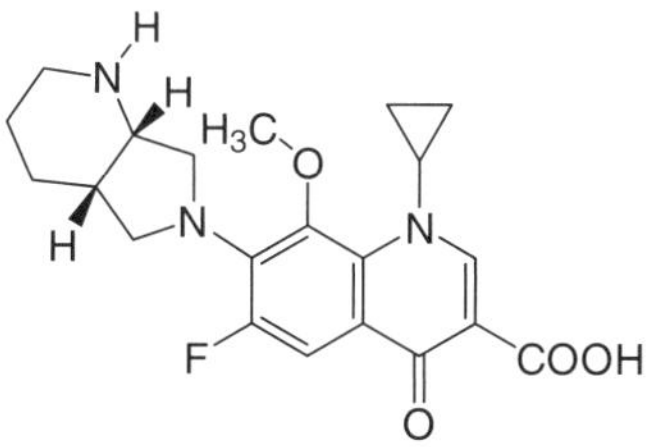

Moxifloxacin

8-6

similar to the antibacterial agent trimethoprim regarding antibacterial spectra, without showing any other similarity regarding chemical structure or mechanism of action.

Norfloxacin is a standard remedy for both lower- and higher-level urinary tract infections. It should be mentioned that quinolones are absorbed rapidly and completely after oral intake, and that they are concentrated in and excreted with the urine, where 10 to 15% of the dose given is to be found in an active form and at a concentration that gives a good antibacterial effect in the urinary tract. Norfloxacin is also a good prophylactic agent against infections with gram-negative enterobacteria in patients with granulocytopenia. Norfloxacin has no effect against streptococci but is effective against gonococci. Gonorrhea infections can be treated by a single 800-mg dose of norfloxacin.

Ciprofloxacin has a broad antibacterial spectrum which includes most of the clinically important pathogens. With them it shows even lower MIC values than that of norfloxacin. Its largest effect is against gram-negative rods, but gram-positive cocci such as streptococci and staphylococci show an intermediate susceptibility. Ciprofloxacin is very effective against typhoid fever and other septic *Salmonella* infections, that is, *Salmonella* infections penetrating the bloodstream. Treatment with ciprofloxacin and other quinolones is the only alternative, with oral administration for infections with *Pseudomonas aeruginosa*. With increasing resistance to traditionally used antibacterial agents against *Mycobacterium tuberculosis* (Chapter 9), quinolones have also become important remedies in the treatment of tuberculosis and can substantially shorten the multidrug treatment regimens for this disease. Ciprofloxacin is one of the most commonly used antibacterial agents in the world. About a decade ago ciprofloxacin acquired doubtful fame when American civil servants lined up to get this remedy (Cipro) for prophylaxis against anthrax disease, which terrorists threatened to spread to federal authorities through letters containing spores of *Bacillus anthracis*. Ofloxacin, levofloxacin, and moxifloxacin have antibacterial spectra similar to those of norfloxacin and ciprofloxacin.

BACTERIAL RESISTANCE TO QUINOLONES

Today unfortunately, pathogenic bacteria often show resistance to quinolones. This resistance appears in three forms. The most common and explainable form is caused by spontaneous mutations hitting the target structure: first, those genes that express the gyrase protein, and second, the gene expressing topoisomerase IV. Spontaneous mutations would change the protein to lower its affinity for the inhibiting quinolone. A second form of resistance is efflux; that is, the resistant bacterium has acquired a mechanism that while spending energy is able to pump the quinolone out of the bacterial cell. This is comparable to the tetracycline resistance described in Chapter 7. The third mechanism of resistance was quite unexpectedly relatively recently found to be plasmid-borne.

Mutational Resistance

Spontaneous mutations in those genes expressing gyrase and topoisomerase IV, respectively, can be calculated to occur at a frequency of 10^{-9} to 10^{-10} per generation. This can be looked at as a very low frequency, but as a consequence, under the powerful selection pressure of a very large consumption of quinolones, it has led to widespread resistance with clinical difficulties in treating infections. As mentioned earlier, the gyrase enzyme consists of four pairwise identical subunits to form a tetramer (A_2B_2). The two A subunits are responsible for cutting the DNA double strand and religating the subunits in the overtwinning reaction (see Fig. 8.1). In the well-characterized A subunit there is a specific area around serine 83 that has been shown to be critical for binding the inhibiting quinolone. Mutationally resistant bacteria show one or several amino acid changes in the area between amino acid residues 67 and 106. Certain pathogens, such as *Campylobacter jejuni, Klebsiella pneumoniae*, and *Pseudomonas aeruginosa*, have a threonine instead of serine at position 83, leaving them with a tenfold lower susceptibility to quinolones than that of bacteria with serine at position 83. It could be surmised that the more bulky threonine molecule interferes with optimal binding of the inhibiting quinolone.

Resistance by Quinolone Efflux

Proteins located in the cytoplasmic membrane of bacteria, efflux proteins, have the ability to pump out toxic substances from the cell against a concentration gradient at a cost in energy. Efflux proteins of this type can effect quinolone resistance. This could be compared to the mechanism of tetracycline resistance, where a specific protein in the bacterial cytoplasmic membrane pumps out tetracycline from the bacterial cell (Chapter 7). The pathogen *P. aeruginosa* could be mentioned as an example of this type of quinolone resistance. This pathogen has been shown to overproduce earlier known efflux proteins (Mex proteins) by a mutationally changed regulation, resulting in resistance to several antibacterial agents, including quinolones. In strains of *P. aeruginosa*, which are quinolone resistant by the efflux mechanism, an increased transcription of several genes for efflux proteins has been observed in the form of increased concentrations of mRNA from these genes.

Transferable Plasmid-Borne Resistance

Single reports on plasmid-borne resistance to quinolones were published in the mid-1980s, but the observations in them were never verified and a mechanism could not be defined. Transferable quinolone resistance was long held to be impossible from a biological point of view. This opinion was based on the knowledge available on mechanisms of plasmid-borne resistance to antibacterial agents. Quinolones are completely synthetic and unnatural substances that could not be imagined as substrates for degrading or modifying enzymes originating in living organisms, finally ending up in pathogens under the selection pressure of a large quinolone distribution, all in analogy with, for example, betalactamases and chloramphenicol acetyl transferases. It should be noted that quinolones are notoriously stable and could be regarded as an environmental threat if spread in the soil of arable land. Furthermore, intracellularly quinolone susceptibility is dominant over quinolone resistance. This means that a plasmid-borne gene *gyr*A (expressing the gyrase A subunit), changed mutationally not to bind quinolones, would not mediate quinolone resistance to a bacterial cell if introduced into it, for example, by conjugation. Such a cell would certainly hold a quinolone-resistant A protein expressed from the plasmid, but it would also contain quinolone-binding, quinolone-susceptible *gyr*A protein expressed from the chromosome, which according to the mechanism of quinolone action would induce DNA damage.

It can be surmised that only a very small number of DNA lesions of this type per cell are sufficient for an antibacterial effect. All these considerations contributed to a sort of consensus that plasmid-borne and transferable quinolone resistance could not exist. But at the end of the 1990s, to the great surprise of all microbiologists, plasmid-borne and conjugatable quinolone resistance was demonstrated irrefutably. The original finding was in a clinical isolate of *K. pneumoniae* from a urinary culture observed in a clinical laboratory in Birmingham, Alabama. A few years later the similarly astonishing mechanism of resistance was defined. With an anthropomorphic view this could be viewed as the microbiological world outwitting all those dead-certain microbiologists. Bacteria are older and wiser than we. It can also be said that the most interesting and trail-blazing discoveries are astonishing, and it is significant that reports about those discoveries often begin: "To our great surprise . . . ".

The mechanism of plasmid-borne quinolone resistance investigated was shown to involve a gene together with other genes expressing antibiotics resistance on a rather large conjugatable plasmid. Experiments demonstrated that the quinolone resistance could be transferred to and expressed in several other enterobacteria, such as E. coli, and also in Pseudomonas. The gene was denoted qnr for quinolone resistance and was shown to be located in an integronlike context upstream of qacE and sul1 (see Chapter 10). Both its plasmid localization and its integron context imply the great ability of the quinolone resistance gene to spread among bacteria. Systematic surveys of clinical isolates have also shown that the qnr gene is spread widely among E. coli, K. pneumoniae, and in enterobacteria in general in the United States, Europe, and China.

The quinolone resistance gene expresses a peptide of 218 amino acids, which was able to protect DNA gyrase from the inhibiting effect of quinolones by binding to the enzyme and thus disallowing the drug from binding to it. By measuring E. coli DNA gyrase activity in the test tube it was shown that purified qnr protein could protect the enzyme from the inhibiting effect of ciprofloxacin. The protecting effect was proportional to the concentration of qnr protein added. It was also shown that the protecting effect was abolished if the qnr protein was denatured by boiling before it was added.

By comparisons of amino acid sequences, the resistance protein expressed from qnr was shown to belong to a known family of proteins, characterized by pentapeptide repetitions (i.e., its members show repetitions of a motif of five amino acids). Proteins of that type have been observed in many different bacterial species. One such protein is McbgG, a component of a system protecting microcin B17 bacteria from intoxicating themselves. Microcin B17 is an antibacterial peptide with an effect similar to that of ciprofloxacin. A certain degree of quinolone resistance has also been demonstrated in bacteria carrying a plasmid-borne gene for McbgG. Similar proteins have also been observed in *Bacillus subtilis, Enterococcus faecalis*, and *Mycobacterium tuberculosis*. These observations could be interpreted to mean that the specific *qnr* protein ought to be found in this group of proteins. Rather recently there was a report describing a systematic search for the *qnr* gene among gram-negative bacterial species by DNA sequence comparisons. This search resulted in the finding in *Shewanella algae* of a gene identical to that found originally on a plasmid in *K. pneumoniae* The *S. algae* is a sea-living pathogenic bacterium that causes infections related to exposure to seawater, suggesting that seawater can be regarded as a reservoir for antibiotic resistance genes.

Further studies on proteins similar to that from *qnr*A, as the first gene found has been denoted, and in particular their three-dimensional structure, have shown a similarity to the structure of DNA. In one of these studies a *qnr*-like protein was isolated from *M. tuberculosis*, as mentioned earlier, and in quantities large enough for x-ray crystallographic studies. The repeated pentapeptides were shown to form a right-hand spiral with a diameter comparable to that of DNA. Further structural studies in silico with virtual models produced by a computer could show that the *qnr*-like protein fitted precisely into the active center of the gyrase enzyme, forming a protein–protein complex, excluding both DNA and quinolones. It should be added here that quinolones bind to the normal gyrase–DNA complex, not to the gyrase alone.

Test tube experiments showed, furthermore, that the *qnr*A-like protein inhibited the gyrase function. This probably leads to slower bacterial growth, but for the bacterium, this is better than to be killed by the quinolone. This argument can be turned around further to the possibility of finding or synthesizing a small molecule with properties analogous to those of the *qnr* protein to stop the growth of bacteria. That could lead to much-needed new antibacterial agents. After defining the concept of plasmid-borne quinolone resistance, and characterization of the *qnr*A gene, several resistance genes of this type have been found. At a food-mediated eruption of *Shigella flexneri* infections in Japan in 2003, a plasmid-borne gene for quinolone resistance was found and named *qnr*S. Its corresponding amino acid sequence shows a 59% amino acid sequence identity with the corresponding sequence of *qnr*A. The origin of *qnr*S is not known. Still another transferable quinolone resistance gene *qnr*B was found in a clinical isolate of *K. pneumoniae* from the southern part of India. Its corresponding amino acid sequence is about 40% identical to that of the *qnr*A. Furthermore, an isolate of *E. coli* recently isolated in the United States hosted a close relative to *qnr*B, differing by only five amino acids from the *qnr*B protein found originally. The origin of *qnr*B is not known. All these observations seem to mean that quinolone resistance will soon be very widespread. All the *qnr* proteins mentioned have the pentapeptide structure described earlier.

It should be added here that another type of plasmid-borne quinolone resistance has already been mentioned in Chapter 6. That was the mutationally changed enzyme of aminoglycoside acetyltransferase, in which spontaneous mutations had changed the substrate spectrum of the enzyme to include a quinolone, ciprofloxacin. That was a notable development under the intense increase in the medical use of ciprofloxacin: A single-function resistance enzyme crossed substrate group boundaries to become capable of mediating resistance to unrelated antimicrobial agents, one of which is fully synthetic and which has not been present in nature until its relatively recent medical use.

Finally, *qnr*-like genes, expressing DNA-like proteins, have been found not only in several bacterial species, but also in fruit flies and in humans. They seem to have a general biological function, which could be speculated to be involvement in the regulation of DNA-binding proteins and of cellular growth.

CONCLUSION

Plasmid-borne resistance against quinolones mediated by *qnr* genes is a clear example of the extraordinary ability of bacteria to adapt to those environmental changes that our use of antibiotics has meant to the microbial world. Finding the *qnr* protein in human pathogens also demonstrates the efficiency of those genetic mechanisms transporting resistance genes horizontally over long biological distances. In the case of *qnr* proteins, these seem basically to be involved in the regulation of DNA synthesis and have here been adapted to a new and artificial function in protecting bacteria from synthetic quinolones. Those genetic transport mechanisms might also have been developed and selected for by our distribution of antibiotics (see Chapter 10).

CHAPTER 9

ANTIBACTERIAL AGENTS NOT RELATED TO THE LARGE ANTIBIOTIC FAMILIES

Agents against tuberculosis are described here as well as nitrofurantoin and phosphomycin. These drugs are now used less as antibacterial agents in urinary tract infections. Finally, nitroimidazoles, which have found use against the peptic ulcer bacterium *Helicobacter pylori*, are discussed.

REMEDIES FOR TUBERCULOSIS

The tuberculosis bacillus belongs to the bacterial family of mycobacteria, microbials that are a living part of soil. There is evidence to show that mycobacteria emerged from the soil to find a niche first infesting, then infecting, various mammals and birds. *Mycobacterium bovis* is a common animal pathogen affecting a variety of animals, including ruminants and primates. It has been speculated that the tuberculosis bacterium was introduced into humankind when humans domesticated cattle some 7000 years ago. Genetic analysis has demonstrated that *M. bovis* and *Mycobacterium tuberculosis* are virtually the same species.

Antibiotics and Antibiotics Resistance, First Edition. Ola Sköld.
© 2011 John Wiley & Sons, Inc. Published 2011 by John Wiley & Sons, Inc.

The bovine bacterium has, however, limited disease-producing capacity in humans, within which it has subtly undergone host adaptation to emerge as the tuberculosis bacillus, *M. tuberculosis*. The disease of tuberculosis has been rampant in Europe and North America for the past five centuries. During the seventeenth and eighteenth centuries "the white plague" took the life of one in five humans in these parts of the world. In the years 1850–1950, before medical treatment was introduced, 1 billion persons are estimated to have died from the disease. The tuberculosis bacterium turned out to be highly resistant to the first selectively acting antibacterial agents, such as the sulfonamides and penicillin. However, a betalactam derivative, meropenem, has recently been shown to have an effect on *M. tuberculosis*, particularly in combination with clavulanic acid (see later in the chapter). As mentioned in Chapter 6, streptomycin was the first selectively acting agent that could be used to treat tuberculosis. The severe side effects were also described. They are so severe that streptomycin is no longer used against tuberculosis. Instead, today four standard remedies are used in the treatment of tuberculosis: rifampicin, isoniazid, pyrazinamide, and ethambutol. Of these, rifampicin is the most important. A few other drugs for the treatment of tuberculosis are also mentioned later in the chapter. The antibacterial treatment of tuberculosis takes a long time because of the growth properties of *M. tuberculosis* and because of the infectious characteristics of the disease. It takes several months to carry through. Because of this long time, mutational resistance becomes a great threat. Because of this risk it becomes very important to treat the infection with several antibacterial agents given in combination at the same time. Random bacterial mutations leading to resistance to individual drugs occur infrequently during bacterial replication, approximately once in 10^5 to 10^8 replications, and the resistance mutations to different drugs are unlinked. The probability of the spontaneous mutational resistance to two drugs is then the product of two mutational probabilities, that is, roughly 1 in $10^5 \times 1$ in $10^6 = 1$ in 10^{11}. The number of bacilli in a patient, also with extensive disease, rarely exceeds 10^9, which means that the occurrence of multiresistant mutants is highly improbable. The combination of drugs then means that the multiplication of low mutational resistance frequencies results in a much lower risk for antibacterial resistance.

Rifampicin

With the example of many antibiotics found earlier in soil microorganisms, a group of compounds, the rifamycins (**9-1**), which have an antibacterial effect, were found at the end of the 1950s in the soil bacterium *Streptomyces mediterranei*. These substances were shown to belong to a chemical group called *ansa compounds*. The structure of these compounds contains an aromatic ring system, naphtokinone, over which there is a long aliphatic carbon bridge. That long bridge gives an impression of a handle (*ansa* in Greek; see **9-1**). The rifamycins bear no similarity to any other antibiotic of medical use. With the purpose of finding useful antimicrobial remedies, medicinal chemists have synthesized many rifamycin variants, among

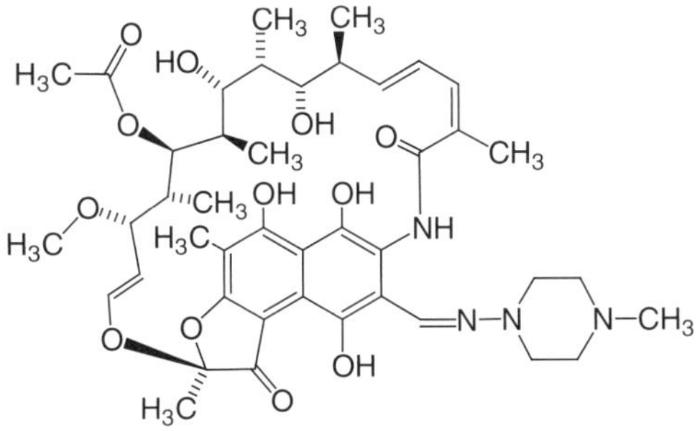

Rifampicin

9-1

them a piperazin derivative, rifampicin, which in oral administration provides a very good antibacterial effect.

Rifampicin has a broad antibacterial spectrum, although gram-negative rods such as *E. coli* are less susceptible. This is because the large molecule cannot very well penetrate the thick lipopolysacharide layer of these bacteria. Rifampicin is, however, very effective against *M. tuberculosis* and is a first-choice remedy in the treatment of tuberculosis. Rifampicin is also very effective against both gram-positive and gram-negative cocci and has found good use with severe and hard-to-handle staphylococcal infections. Also, with infectious meningitis caused by *Neisseria meningitidis*, rifampicin has found good use for both treatment and prophylaxis. Rifampicin is also at present a first-choice remedy for the treatment of leprosy.

Mechanism of Action

Rifampicin interferes with the growth of bacteria by inhibiting the transcription of DNA, particularly transcriptional initiation. At experiments in vitro with RNA polymerase from *E. coli* the transcription reaction is inhibited to 50% at rifampicin concentrations as low as 2×10^{-8} M. The inhibition is effected by the binding of rifampicin to the DNA transcribing enzyme RNA polymerase. This is a large and complex enzyme, which in bacteria comprises five peptide subunits, one of which occurs in a pair. The complete enzyme, the holoenzyme, is built of two alpha subunits, one beta subunit, one beta' subunit, and one sigma subunit. (For further details, see textbooks on biochemistry and bacterial genetics.) The active center of the beta subunit catalyzes the polymerization, and this is where rifampicin binds to inhibit the polymerization activity. The corresponding enzyme in mammalian cells does not bind rifampicin, which is then acting selectively on bacteria.

Resistance

Unfortunately, resistance toward rifampicin is common. It arises easily by spontaneous mutations in the bacterial gene expressing the beta subunit of RNA polymerase, which then loses its affinity for the drug. The common occurrence of rifampicin resistance is explained partially by the nucleotide composition of the beta subunit gene, which is unusually A-T rich, which makes it prone to spontaneous mutations. This resistance development threatens the treatment of tuberculosis, for which, as noted, rifampicin is a very important remedy. The mutationally induced rifampicin resistance in *M. tuberculosis* can be determined quickly by polymerase chain reaction. Resistance determination would otherwise be very difficult to handle because of the very slow growth of the tuberculosis bacterium. These conditions of resistance necessitate the combination of rifampicin with other antibacterial agents in tuberculosis treatment, which has to continue for several months. The combination of several antibacterial agents means that the low frequencies of spontaneous mutations to resistance for each agent are multiplied by one another, resulting in a very low probability of simultaneous mutation toward resistance to two or more antibacterial agents.

Plasmid-Borne Resistance

Transferable plasmid-borne resistance to rifampicin was long regarded as nonexistent. During the 1990s, however, integron cassettes (see Chapter 10) were observed to mediate rifampicin resistance in clinical isolates of, for example, *Pseudomonas aeruginosa* and *E. coli*. Integron-borne genes can transfer with transposons and with plasmids and then also horizontally between bacteria (see Chapter 10). The mechanism of this rifampicin resistance was shown to consist of an enzyme that inactivates rifampicin by transferring an ADP-ribosyl molecule to one of the hydroxyl groups of the long aliphatic carbon chain (*ansa*) of the rifampicin structure (see **9-1**). Rifampicin resistance by ribosylation was first characterized in the nontuberculous bacterium *Mycobacterium smegmatis*, which is endogenously resistant to rifampicin. The ribosylating enzyme could be speculated to have evolved as a defense against rifamycins in the microbial world of soil. Its corresponding gene *arr*-1 is located on the chromosome of *M. smegmatis*. A variant of *arr*-1 with a very similar nucleotide sequence, *arr*-2, has been found as an integron cassette (Chapter 10) in pathogenic clinical isolates of *P. aeruginosa* and *E. coli*, both with an origin in southern Asia. The finding of identical *arr*-2 in both *Pseudomonas* and *Escherichia* implies the ability of the integron cassette to move between species. Closer studies of the enzymatic rifampicin inactivation has shown that the enzyme protein expressed from *arr*-2 catalyzes transfer of the ADP-ribose part of NADH to a hydroxyl residue of the aliphatic carbon chain of rifampicin. NADH is the common coenzyme nicotinamide-adenine dinucleotide, which occurs in all living cells. It could be speculated that soil-living *Pseudomonas* could have taken up *arr*-1 from mycobacteria and then transferred it to pathogenic *Pseudomonas*-species in which *arr*-1 developed into *arr*-2 under the selection pressure of rifampicin used clinically. The inclusion of *arr*-2 in an integron cassette has meant a pronounced movability between the genomes of bacteria, including transposons and plasmids, and further between different bacterial species.

Other Agents Against Tuberculosis

In addition to rifampicin there is a semisynthetic derivative of rifamycin, rifabutine, with about the same antibacterial spectrum as rifampicin but which could also have a certain effect against rifampicin-resistant strains of *M. tuberculosis*, showing that cross resistance between rifampicin and rifabutine is not absolute.

Isoniazid or Isonicotinic Acid Hydrazide

Isoniazid (**9-2**) is a specific agent against tuberculosis that has been used for this purpose since 1952, when its remedial properties were recognized after having been characterized as a chemical compound in 1912. It is used in several fixed combinations with rifampicin and with other tuberculostatic drugs, such as pyrazinamide and ethambutol (see later in the chapter). It is used to counteract the development of resistance according to the general arguments given earlier in the chapter, as well as for rifampicin resistance. Isoniazid works very specifically against *M. tuberculosis* and closely related bacteria. The tuberculosis bacterium is extremely sensitive to isoniazid, which shows MIC values of 0.02 to 0.06 μg/mL. To exercise its effect, it has to be activated to isonicotinic acid (**9-3**) in the bacterial cell. This activation is effected by a mycobacteria-specific catalase-peroxidase, which normally protects the bacterial cell against peroxides by degrading them to free oxygen and water but which also seems to be able to oxidize isoniazid to its active form. The oxidized

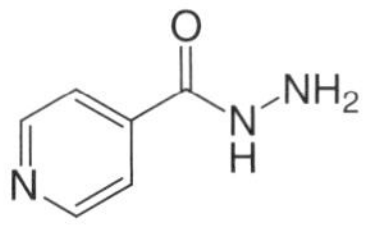

Isoniazide

9-2

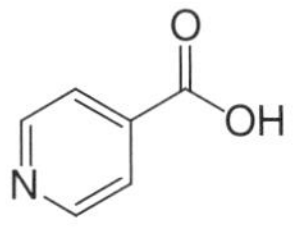

Isonicotinic acid

9-3

active form is thought to work by inhibiting one of the enzymes (InhA) involved in the synthesis of mycolic acids, which are long-chain alpha-branched, beta-hydroxylated fatty acids comprising an important component of the cell wall of the tuberculosis bacterium and which participate in its pathogenic effect against pulmonary tissue.

Resistance against isoniazid occurs and is a threat to treatment, since the lowered susceptibility to one of the components of the drug combination therapy affects the total therapeutic effect and could contribute to the development of multiresistance (see Chapter 10). Isoniazid resistance could be caused by mutations in the *kat*G gene expressing the catalase-peroxidase enzyme, inactivating its enzymic effect and thus preventing it from activating to its antibacterially active form any isoniazid administered. Another form of isoniazid resistance, caused by spontaneous mutations in the gene expressing the mycolic acid–synthesizing enzyme, has been observed. This enzyme is the target of the activated form of isoniazid, and the mutations make it less susceptible to the drug.

Pyrazinamide

Another specifically acting tuberculostatic agent, pyrazinamide (**9-4**), is often used in a fixed combination with rifampicin. The exact mechanism of action for this drug is not known, but it has been shown that it must be converted enzymically inside the cell to pyrazinoic acid (**9-5**), which is the active antibacterial agent.

Pyrazinamide

9-4

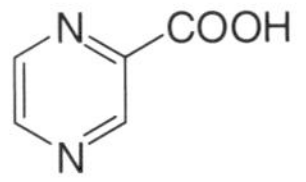

Pyrazinoic acid

9-5

The enzyme responsible for this conversion is pyrazine amidase, and as expected, pyrazinamide-resistant forms of *M. tuberculosis* lack the effect of this enzyme or show its lowered activity. The logical solution to this clinical resistance problem would then be to use pyrazinoic acid as a tuberculostatic drug. Compared to pyrazinamide, however, pyrazinoic acid is taken up very poorly in the bacterial cell.

Ethambutol

The ethylenediamine derivative ethambutol (**9-6**) is another agent used as a component in fixed tuberculostatic drug combinations containing, for example, rifampicin, isoniazide, and pyrazinamide. Ethambutol is a specific tuberculostatic drug which has been used for this purpose since the beginning of the 1960s. It should always be combined with another tuberculostatic drug. Ethambutol has a somewhat wider antibacterial spectrum than isonicotinic acid hydrazide and is also effective against *Mycobacterium avium*, which is an opportunistic pathogen found in AIDS patients. Despite many years of clinical use of ethambutol, its mechanism of action has not been known until relatively recently. It has been shown that ethambutol interferes with

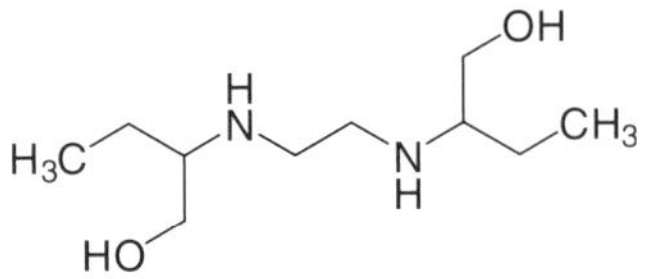

Ethambutol

9-6

the enzymatic system, which in mycobacteria polymerizes the monosacharide arabinose to the polysaccharide that is part of the mycobacterium-specific cell wall component lipoarabinoman-nan. The ethambutol-mediated interference with mycobacterial cell wall formation is regarded as being able to increase the permeability for other antimycobacterial agents and thus contribute to that valuable clinical synergism, observed for example at the combination of ethambutol with rifampicin, which is a large molecule whose size interferes with permeability. Resistance to ethambutol has been observed, and was in many cases, but not all, shown to be caused by spontaneously occurring mutational changes in the synthesis regulation of the enzymes involved in the polymerization of arabinose.

Cycloserine

Cycloserine was used as a remedy against tuberculosis, but is not used much clinically nowadays because of the central nervous system disturbances that were sometimes experienced by patients. It is mentioned here because of its interesting microbiological effect. It is a true antibiotic in the sense that it was originally isolated from several *Streptomyces* species, among them *S. lavendulae*, under the name *oxamycin*. D-Cycloserine (**9-7**) has a simple chemical configuration and is a structural analog of D-alanine. D-Cycloserine is a broad-spectrum antibiotic with a particularly good effect on mycobacteria, among them *M. tuberculosis*. Its microbiological effect is directed against the formation

D-Cycloserine

9-7

of the D-alanine-D-alanyl end of the glucopeptide involved in the final steps of murein synthesis at cell wall formation (see Chapter 4). Two enzymes are involved in the synthesis of this dipeptide. One is L-alanine racemase, forming D-alanine from L-alanine; the other is D-alanine-D-alanine synthetase. Both of these enzymes are inhibited competitively by D-cycloserine. It should be mentioned that D-cycloserine has a 100-fold higher affinity for D-alanine-D-alanine synthetase than does the normal D-alanine substrate. Added D-alanine and L-alanine reverse the inhibitory effect of D-cycloserine. The final effect of D-cycloserine is similar to that of betalactams, of glycopeptides, and also of phosphomycin, in that the bacterium affected is unable to form the crucial transpeptidase cross-links for murein stability and thus for a stable cell wall. Affected bacterial cells will succumb to morphological aberrations and lysis.

Resistance to D-cycloserine occurs frequently. It is caused by spontaneous mutations in the genes expressing L-alanine racemase and D-alanine-D-alanine synthetase to lower the affinity of D-cycloserine for these enzymes. Also, changes in the alanine permease transporting D-cycloserine into the cell have been shown to mediate resistance to the drug. Finally, we note that the side effect of D-cycloserine causing disturbances in the central nervous system has recently been turned into an advantage in that when it is administered as a drug, it functions as an adjuvant to cognitive behavioral therapy in the treatment of obsessive-compulsive disorder.

para-Aminosalicylic Acid

p-Aminosalicylic acid (**9-8**) is a simple substance used earlier as a tuberculostatic remedy. It works as an analog of *p*-aminobenzoic acid and inhibits folic acid synthesis in *M. tuberculosis*, analogous to how sulfonamides work in other bacteria. It was actually p-aminosalicylic acid

9-8

tested as a tuberculostatic drug in 1944, that is, before the use of streptomycin. It has been used as a standard remedy since 1946, often in combination with streptomycin mitigating the selection of resistance against the latter. It must be given in rather large doses, such as 2 to 4 g four times a day. There are side effects such as nausea, vomiting, and diarrhea. Also, hepatitis has been observed as a side effect. Because of the side effects mentioned, and because of its limited efficiency, it has generally been outcompeted by the more recent antibacterials described earlier in the chapter. It is, however, still used in cases of multidrug-resistant disease.

Tuberculostatic Drugs Recruited from Earlier Known Groups of Antibiotics Found Originally with Other Antibacterial Spectra

As mentioned earlier, penicillins were very early found to have no activity against *M. tuberculosis*. It was recently shown that this is due to the rapid hydrolysis of betalactams by the betalactamase produced from the chromosomal *blaC* gene in the tuberculosis bacterium (see also Chapter 4). Experiments in vitro with laboratory strains of *M. tuberculosis*, including strains showing extensive drug resistance, demonstrated a good inhibitory effect of meropenem, particularly when combined with clavulanic acid (Chapter 4). Meropenem, which belongs to the group of carbapenems known for their stability toward betalactamases, showed MIC values of about 1 μg/mL in combination with clavulanic acid toward laboratory strains of *M. tuberculosis*.

Diarylquinolines

The diarylquinolines (**9-9**) differ from both fluoroquinolones and other quinoline classes. One member of this group has a spectrum of potent and selective antimycobacterial activity in vitro. This antibacterial activity includes several drug-resistant strains of *M. tuberculosis*, including strains resistant to fluoroquinolone. This substance shows a MIC value of 0.06 μg/mL with *M. tuberculosis* and shows about 10-fold higher bactericidal activity than isoniazid and rifampicin against this bacterium. The mechanism of action seems to be the inhibition of the proton pump of adenosine triphosphate synthase.

TMC 207, R 207910 (Diarylquinoline)

9-9

Finally, it should be noted that moxifloxacin, which is a fluoroquinolone (see Chapter 8), has been tested successfully against *M. tuberculosis* in animal experiments and in combination with rifampicin and pyrazinamide.

The Battle Against Tuberculosis

The remedies mentioned, together with social measures, have been very successful in limiting tuberculosis in the Western world. The specialized hospitals (sanatoria) and clinics that were widely available throughout the industrialized nations in the

1950s and 1960s have largely been closed. Since humans are the only host for *M. tuberculosis*, there was the hope that the tuberculosis disease could eventually be eradicated. The hope of such a development vanished with the occurrence of two things: drug resistance and HIV. Although the original need for 24 months of drug therapy could be reduced to six months, irregular or incomplete compliance with the regime became an increasing problem. As a consquence of this, the prevalence of drug-resistant strains of *M. tuberculosis* has increased dramatically in certain regions and populations. As an example, in some social contexts in New York City, where a combination of poverty and narcotics abuse has led to deteriorating tuberculosis control, a 33% frequency of cases of resistance to at least one drug was observed, and 19% of the cases were resistant to two or more agents.

In some developing countries, where resources are limited, drug resistance rates of more than 30% have been observed. This development has occurred because patients either discontinue taking one or more of their multiple drugs or take less than the prescribed dose. It could also be that today's physicians, who are less familiar with tuberculosis, prescribe inappropriately. Insufficient amounts of antibacterials are administered, creating an environment that selects for the survival of drug-resistant mutants. This drug resistance development has led to situations where no remedy is active for treatment, termed extensively drug-resistant tuberculosis. Furthermore, the HIV epidemic afflicts persons from socioeconomic groups in which tuberculosis is highly prevalent. Because HIV infects and kills the cell that is central to tuberculosis immunity, the helper T-lymphocyte (CD_4^+), the viral epidemic has led to a dramatic increase in the number of tuberculosis cases in many groups of people in many parts of the world. There are also many examples of the nosocomial spread of multidrug-resistant tuberculosis in highly lethal epidemics among HIV-infected/AIDS patients.

NITROFURANTOIN

The synthetical antibacterial agent nitrofurantoin (**9-10**) has been used for more than 30 years in the treatment of bacterial urinary tract infections. Known by the name Furadantin, it has a broad antibacterial spectrum covering both gram-positive and gram-negative bacteria. It is, however, not active against *Pseudomonas aeruginosa*. It has a good effect against *E. coli* infecting the urinary tract. Side effects in the form of allergic symptoms have increased in frequency, leading to decreased use of the drug. In the cell, bacterial nitroreductases transform nitrofurantoin into several very reactive electrophile derivatives reacting with nucleophile loci in many bacterial macromolecules. Relatively recent studies performed with radioactively labeled nitrofurantoin seemed to show binding to specific ribosomal proteins, suggesting inhibition of protein synthesis. Nitrofurantoin might be looked upon as an inhibitor of ribosomal function, but this interpretation is preliminary and has to be verified. Resistance against nitrofurantoin has not been reported. This could be due to the many points of attack of the reactive nitrofurantoin derivatives.

Nitrofurantoin

9-10

NITROIMIDAZOLES

The two synthetic antibacterial agents metronidazole (**9-11**) and tinidazole (**9-12**) show a good effect against anaerobic bacterial pathogens. One example is the treatment of the much feared enteritis caused by the toxin-producing *Clostridium difficile*. Metronidazole has also found use in the treatment

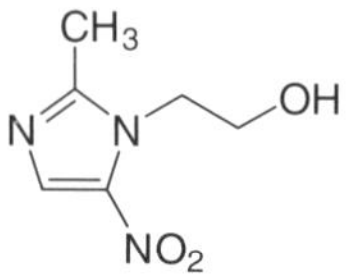

Metronidazole

9-11

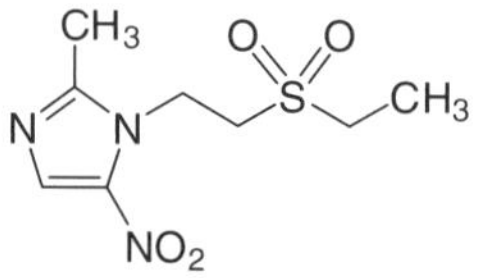

Tinidazole

9-12

of peptic ulcer, since the peptic ulcer bacterium *Helicobacter pylori* is susceptible to this agent. Tinidazole has the same type of use as metronidazole. The selective effect of nitroimidazoles on anaerobic bacteria is dependent on the sufficiently low redox potential of the electron-transferring enzymes of these bacteria to be able to reduce the nitro group of the nitroimidazoles. This initiates the formation of unstable intermediary compounds with effects on bacterial DNA, causing both single and double strand breaks.The precise mechanism for this is not known, but the effect is directed particularly toward the pyrimidine residues of the DNA. The total effect is inhibition of bacterial DNA replication and transcription. Bacterial mutants that are deficient in their DNA repair system are particularly sensitive to nitroimidazoles. The nitroimidazole effect of initiating DNA damage could make them suspicious as potential cancerogenous substances. Mammalian cells (e.g., human cells), however, have a redox potential that is so high that these cells cannot activate nitroimidazoles to form the DNA-damaging metabolites. Metronidazole and other nitroimidazoles can be exonerated from any serious side effect of this type.

Resistance to metronidazole and other nitroimidazoles is due to the diminished ability of the anaerobic bacterial cell to activate the drugs according to the enzymic reactions described. This decreased ability is in turn caused by mutational damage to the nitro group–reducing enzymes. A total loss of these enzymes would result in total resistance to metronidazole, but since they are also vital for bacterial survival, only intermediate resistance is observed.

PHOSPHOMYCIN

A simple phosphonic acid structure, phosphomycin (**9-13**) is an antibacterial agent with a good effect against both gram-positive and gram-negative pathogenic bacteria. A biosynthetic pathway for the formation of phosphomycin has been described in *Streptomyces wedmorensis*, and phosphomycin can thus be regarded as an antibiotic in the true sense of the word. Phosphomycin has had a wide distribution as an antibacterial drug in Spain, Italy, France, and Japan, where it has been used particularly for the treatment of patients with infections in the lower urinary tract. In many other countries it has come to be used very rarely, however. It is described here in some detail because particularly the transferable plasmid-borne resistance to it is very interesting from a microbiological point of view.

The mechanism of action of phosphomycin is distantly similar to that of betalactams. It interferes with bacterial cell wall synthesis, but at a very early stage, where the small molecular element, the glucopeptide, is formed before finally being

Phosphomycin

9-13

incorporated into the mucopolysaccharide of the cell wall. The bacterial cell wall can be viewed as a giant molecule, murein, which has to grow continuously outside the plasma membrane by bacterial growth. For this to take place, the monomer of the polysaccharide, the glycopeptide, has to be synthesized inside the cell and then transported out through the cytoplasmic membrane borne on an isoprene derivative, bactoprenole, which could pass through the lipid cell membrane. One of the early steps in the glycopeptide synthesis is the condensation of the sugar component N-acetyl glucosamine with phosphoenolpyruvate to form the lactyl residue to which the pentapeptide of the glucopeptide is attached. (For biochemical details, see the cell wall chapter of a microbiology textbook.) Phosphomycin can be looked upon as a pyruvate analog, inhibiting the condensation which is effected by the enzyme, pyruvate-UDP-N-acetyl glucoseamine transferase. The inhibition takes place by the very reactive epoxy group of phosphomycin binding covalently to one of the cysteine residues of the enzyme.

Resistance against phosphomycin is observed by mutational changes in the transferase enzyme, diminishing its affinity for the drug. Phosphomycin has been shown to be taken up in the cell by the cellular transport systems for glycerophosphate and hexosephosphate, respectively, and mutational changes in these systems could lead to phosphomycin resistance.

Quite unexpectedly, transferable plasmid-borne resistance to phosphomycin has been observed. Unexpectedly, because the small molecule with its specific epoxy structure was thought of as hardly being a substrate for an acquired enzyme to degrade or modify it. As mentioned, phosphomycin has been used widely in Spain, where highly resistant clinical isolates showed up. Most of these were due to spontaneous chromosomal mutations hitting the functions of glucopeptide formation and cellular uptake. However, in gram-negative nosocomial strains of *Serratia marcescens*, for example, transferable plasmid-borne high resistance toward phosphomycin was found. It turned out that the resistance-mediating plasmid carried a gene expressing glutathion-*S*-transferase with the ability to catalyze a reaction between the sulfhydryl group of the glutathione cysteine and the epoxy group of phosphomycin to form a covalent bond inactivating the antibacterial effect of phosphomycin.

The glutathione transferase has been characterized biochemically and its corresponding gene sequenced. The gene is called *fos*A. Also in gram-positive pathogens such as *Staphylococcus epidermidis* and *S. aureus*, plasmid-borne resistance to phosphomycin was observed to be effected by the same transferase mechanism. The nucleotide sequence of the corresponding gene was different, however; called *fos*B, its expressed amino acid sequence showed 50% identity with the glutathione transferase expressed from *fos*A. The glutathione transferase from *fos*B also inactivated phosphomycin by forming a covalent bond between the sulfhydryl group of glutathione cysteine and the epoxy group of phosphomycin. It was later observed that on the chromosome of the soil bacterium *Bacillus subtilis* there is a gene whose nucleotide sequence is 63% identical to that of *fos*B. The product of this gene could be viewed as a defense against toxic products in the soil-living organism, parallel to the detoxifying function of glutathione transferase in mammalian cells. The *fos*B-like gene of the soil bacterium could be speculated to have developed into the *fos*A and *fos*B of pathogens under the selection pressure of a large drug distribution. Later, several homologs to *fos*A and *fos*B have been characterized in transposon-borne integron cassettes.

CONCLUSION

Most of the agents treated in this chapter have been tuberculostatic. Tuberculosis is a rather rare disease in today's industrialized world, so the drugs discussed are not distributed very widely in countries with extended health care organizations. Internationally, however, tuberculosis is a commonly occurring disease spreading at an increasing rate. Nitrofurantoin, nitroimidazoles, and phosphomycin have been treated in some detail because their mechanisms of action, and the resistance against them in bacteria, are interesting from a microbiological point of view.

CHAPTER *10*

MECHANISMS FOR THE HORIZONTAL SPREAD OF ANTIBIOTIC RESISTANCE AMONG BACTERIA

In this chapter we describe how pathogenic bacteria can acquire genes that mediate antibiotic resistance and how these genes can spread between bacteria by many different genetic transport mechanisms. There is also a short description of antibiotic resistance by spontaneous mutations.

TRANSFERABLE RESISTANCE: CONJUGATION

In earlier chapters we mentioned that resistance to several antibacterial agents can spread horizontally from bacterium to bacterium, and even promiscuously, in the sense that transfer can also take place between bacterial species. The property of resistance must be represented in the bacterial genome; thus the transfer of resistance must include the transfer of DNA between bacteria, most commonly by the bacterial genetic phenomenon of conjugation (Fig. 10.1). We should note that the particular study of antibiotic resistance and its spread in bacterial populations has

Antibiotics and Antibiotics Resistance, First Edition. Ola Sköld.
© 2011 John Wiley & Sons, Inc. Published 2011 by John Wiley & Sons, Inc.

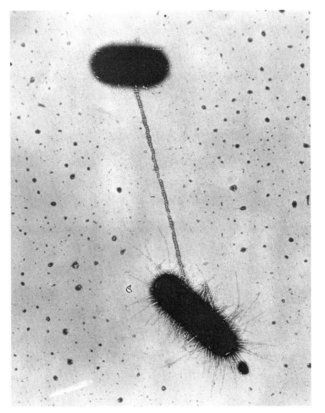

FIGURE 10.1 Bacterial conjugation. Conjugation between cells of *E. coli* as seen in an electron microscope. The pilus of the donor bacterium establishes a cell-to-cell contact between donor and recipient.

played a seminal role in the development of recombinant DNA technology and its applications, and the study of plasmid-borne resistance has granted a very large benefit to basic molecular biological science in general. The transfer of antibiotic resistance between bacteria could be called *contagious resistance*, in that antibiotic-susceptible bacteria are infected with resistance genes. The mechanism of conjugation mentioned has the ability to transfer several resistance genes at the same time, *contagious multiresistance*.

That genetic material could be transferred between bacteria at cell contact was first observed in experiments with *E. coli* in 1946. Those first observations led to the discovery of the F factor (F for fertility), which turned out to be an extrachromosomal genetic element with the ability to transfer from one bacterial cell to another at cell contact. That the latter was essential was obvious from the fact that agitation and blending abolished the transfer. The F (for "fertility") factor was also found to be able to induce the transfer of chromosomal genes from one cell to another, a kind of sexuality to form new gene combinations. For a more detailed description of this very important bacterial phenomenon, see textbooks on microbiology. The F factor is a circular DNA molecule, occurring in small numbers outside the large cellular, circular chromosome. At cell growth the F factor is replicated in phase with the chromosome. Extrachromosomal genetic elements such as the F factor, called *plasmids,* appear in many different forms in the bacterial world. With the F factor as an example, many other plasmids with the ability to transfer from bacterium to bacterium have been identified. This phenomenon of transfer, called *conjugation,* is effected by a proteinaceous fingerlike structure, a pilus, induced by the plasmid and located on the surface of the host bacterium. The pilus can establish contact with another bacterium (see Fig. 10.1).

The discoverers of the conjugation phenomenon described it as a form of bacterial sexuality, but the analogy cannot be extended to pili, which were originally called sex pili. But the pilus does not have a penis function; rather it can be looked upon as an arm with the ability to bind to the surface of a recipient cell, later to be retracted to establish close contact between the two conjugating cells. The DNA molecule transferred probably does not pass through the pilus but through a separate channel that is formed between the two conjugating cells. The plasmid-carrying cell can send the plasmid DNA through this channel to

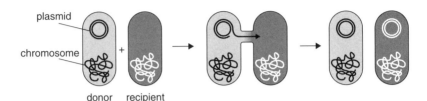

FIGURE 10.2 Schematic illustration of conjugation between bacteria. The leftmost part shows the donor with its transferable plasmid and a recipient bacterium. In the middle part of the figure cell-to-cell contact is established and one strand of the plasmid DNA is on its way into the recipient to replicate. On the right, conjugation is completed, where both the strand left behind by the donor plasmid and the strand transferred have replicated to form complete plasmids in both donor and recipient.

the other cell but not the entire plasmid—only a single strand of the circular double-stranded molecule from the host. The single strand left in the donor cell is replicated to its double-stranded form, and the strand transferred to the recipient cell is replicated. The final result is then that both the donor and the recipient cell end up with one complete plasmid copy each (Fig. 10.2).

MUTATIONAL RESISTANCE

Mutations mediating resistance against many different antibacterial agents by changing antibiotic target structures have been described in earlier chapters. It is important to point out that these mutations are spontaneous and not in any way directed by the antibacterial agent. These mutations occur in that steady stream of genome changes to which all living organisms are subjected. They are caused by replication errors or by DNA changes caused by external agents such as natural radioactivity or cosmic radiation. Spontaneous mutations that happen to mediate a lowered susceptibility to a certain antibacterial agent will then be rapidly selected to dominance in the presence of that particular agent. This is a self-evident consequence of their growth advantage over their nonmutated and susceptible bacterial relatives. That the occurrence of resistance mutations is completely independent of the presence of the growth-inhibiting agent is a fundamental principle of bacterial genetics that was settled in the 1940s.

PLASMID-BORNE RESISTANCE AGAINST ANTIBACTERIAL AGENTS

Sulfonamides were used as antibacterial agents with good results in epidemics of *Shigella* dysentery in Japan in the middle of the 1940s after the end of World War II. The good clinical effect of sulfonamides against those *Shigella* species causing dysentery was not permanent, however. In 1952 more than 80% of the *Shigella* isolates showed a high resistance against sulfonamides. During the 1950s streptomycin, tetracycline, and chloramphenicol were introduced and used frequently in the treatment of *Shigella* dysentery in Japan. Resistance followed with the occurrence of clinical *Shigella* isolates insensitive to tetracycline or streptomycin. In 1956, however, an isolate was found that showed resistance against all four of the antibacterial agents: sulfonamides, tetracycline, streptomycin, and chloramphenicol. Just about a year later this multiresistance against four antibacterial agents was common among clinical *Shigella* isolates. It was conceptually very difficult to explain this clinical resistance phenomenon by referring to mutation and selection, since resistance against sulfonamides, streptomycin, tetracycline, and chloramphenicol is represented by different chromosomal genes as described in earlier chapters. The mutational frequency for a single resistance mutation is about 10^{-7} to 10^{-10} per bacterium and generation, leading to vanishingly small frequencies for multiresistance of the type mentioned. It is possible to think of a rare single *Shigella* strain that could have gone through a mutational development toward multiresistance, but in Japan then, many serologically different *Shigella* strains from different outbreaks of dysentery were observed to show multiresistance of the type described.

Careful epidemiological studies showed unusual clinical conditions in some epidemics. Cultivations of *Shigella* from the same patient could, for example, contain both multiresistant and fully susceptible strains of the same serotype. Certain patients could unexpectedly excrete multiresistant bacteria despite the fact that upon falling ill they excreted only susceptible bacteria and then had been treated with only one antibacterial drug. Such an observation is incompatible with a multiresistance development by accumulated resistance mutations. Furthermore, in one epidemic, strains of *E. coli* could be isolated which showed the same resistance against sulfonamides, streptomycin, chloramphenicol, and tetracyclines as that of the disease-causing *Shigella* strain.

There was no acceptable explanation of these microbiological phenomena until the Japanese bacteriologist Tomoichiro Akiba suggested that the multiresistance could be transferred from resistant strains of *E. coli* to the *Shigella* pathogen in the gastrointestinal canal of the patient. This hypothesis, together with experimental results to support it, was presented at a conference of the Japanese Bacteriological Society in November 1959 and later published in the Japanese Journal of Microbiology. Similar experiments were performed by Kunitaro Ochiai independent of Akiba and presented one day later in November 1959 to the Japanese Society for Chemotherapy and then published in the Japanese Medical Journal in 1959. The simplest experiment that these two Japanese microbiologists performed was to mix multiresistant *E. coli* with susceptible *Shigella* cells in broth, and then by selective cultivation show the appearance of *Shigella* strains with the same pattern of resistance as that of the *E. coli* donor. Corresponding experiments were performed on patients by introducing multiresistant *E. coli* per rectum, then showing uptake in originally susceptible *Shigella* strains of the resistance pattern of the *E. coli* bacteria, demonstrating that resistance transfer took place in the gut of the patient.

Both Tomoichiro Akiba and Kunitaro Ochiai interpreted the resistance transfer phenomenon according to the conjugation principle discovered about 10 years earlier—DNA transfer via cellular contact—and named the transferred resistance properties *R factors*. This interpretation was supported by the experimental observation that the resistance-carrying bacteria could be cured from resistance by treatment with acridine orange, which was known to be able to eliminate an episome, an extrachromosomal genetic element, from a bacterium. The name was later changed to *R plasmid*, which is more in line with present knowledge. Akiba and Ochiai published their results in the Japanese language, which meant that their observations did not become known in the Western world until 1963, when Tsutomu Watanabe published a review article, "Infective Heredity of Multiple Drug Resistance in Bacteria," in *Bacteriological Reviews* (American Society of Microbiology). While this review article was in press in 1962, Naomi Datta in London reported on the appearance of R plasmids in strains of *Salmonella typhimurium* isolated in England. Very soon thereafter, R plasmids were observed all over the world, revealing their great potential for the spread of resistance and the consequences for the medical use of antibiotics.

PLASMIDS

As mentioned earlier, plasmids are extrachromosomal genetic elements in the form of circular DNA molecules replicating outside the bacterial chromosome, but in congruence with its replication. The latter regulatory link is of course very important, since a faster replication would overcrowd the cell with plasmids, and kill it, while a slower replication would very quickly dilute the plasmid away. Bacterial plasmids vary dramatically in size, from a few thousand base pairs to half a million base pairs (0.5 Mb, mega base pairs) or more. According to the argument mentioned earlier, there is a lower limit of plasmid size defined by those genes needed for the regulation of plasmid replication in relation to the chromosome. These genes, together with the replication initiation of the plasmid, comprise what is called a *replicon*. For a more detailed description of the function of these regulatory genes, see textbooks on bacterial genetics.

As mentioned, the transfer and spread of antibiotic resistance genes with R plasmids depend on the conjugation ability of these plasmids. That is the ability to transfer a copy of itself from its host bacterium to a recipient bacterium. Also as mentioned earlier, conjugation depends on contact between bacterial cells via a pilus, pulling donor and recipient together to close cell contact. The mechanism of conjugation requires a substantial amount of genetic space; that is, several genes are needed to express those proteins forming a pilus and those that effect the DNA single-strand transfer from cell to cell. As a simple rule of thumb, the size of this genetic space is about 30 kb (30 kilo base pairs). According to the same simple rule, this means that plasmids below a size of 30 kb cannot conjugate. Small plasmids can all the same transfer from bacterium to bacterium together with larger conjugating plasmids. This phenomenon, called *mobilization*, means that the small plasmid is transferred via the transfer channel that the larger plasmid has formed for its own transfer (Fig. 10.3). Experimentally, it is thus possible to arrange a triple cross, where a small nonconjugatable plasmid is transferred to a recipient. In the first cross, a conjugatable plasmid is transferred to a recipient hosting the small plasmid. In a second cross, the small plasmid is transferred via the transfer channel that the large conjugatable plasmid forms when transferring to a recipient, which at the end will host both plasmids. This is a triple cross—three different host bacteria are involved.

The mobilization phenomenon is limited to certain plasmid classes and related to their characteristics of replication. For

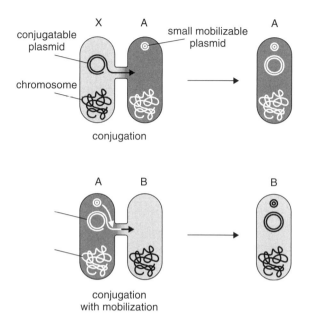

FIGURE 10.3   Small plasmid mobilization. A small nontransferable plasmid is mobilized from one bacterial cell to another with the help of a larger transferable plasmid in a triple cross. In the upper left a large conjugatable plasmid is introduced by conjugation into the bacterium harboring the small nontransferable plasmid. The lower left part illustrates how the large transferable plasmid mobilizes the small plasmid into the final recipient by another conjugation.

further details, see textbooks of bacterial genetics under mobilization. After the original discoveries regarding R plasmids at the beginning of the 1960s, a very large number of R plasmids carrying all sorts of resistance genes have been characterized. They can largely be characterized and classified by the characteristic genes of their replicons. They can be classified in *inc* groups. The name *inc* is derived from the word *incompatibility*, and the classification is based on the inability of different plasmid replicons to exist stably in the same host bacterium, which is in turn related to the characteristics of the corresponding replicon genes. R plasmids as well as replicon genes can carry varying numbers of drug resistance genes. These can reach numbers of 10 or more. An example is the rifampicin-resistance-carrying R plasmid inferred in Chapter 9. Besides rifampicin resistance, this R plasmid carries resistance against betalactams, netilmicin, tobramycin, amikacin, gentamicin, strep-tomycin, spectinomycin, sulfonamides, and chloramphenicol. This means that a pathogenic bacterial strain taking up this plas-mid by conjugation at the same time becomes resistant to 10 antibiotics, and that treatment of an infection with this bacterium using one of these 10 agents also selects for resistance against the other nine.

The very large multitude and variety of both resistance genes and plasmid replicons that has been observed makes it very interesting to ask questions about the origin of R plasmids and their structure. This is the case particularly because it can be surmised that the development of R plasmids has for decades been driven to a large extent by the very large distribution of antibacterial agents in the microbial environment. Three very interesting questions could be discerned: The first regards the origin of the R-plasmid replicons, the second is about the origin of resistance genes, and the third asks about those genetic mech-anisms that have been able to transport resistance genes and to insert them into plasmids.

The Origin of R Plasmids

A very large number of different R plasmids have been observed. In Europe. R plasmids were first observed and characterized by the British bacteriologist Naomi Datta at the beginning of the 1960s. She asked if the great multitude of R plasmids had devel-oped under the selection pressure of our antibiotics. To approach this question, she turned to a collection of enterobacterial isolates which had been collected before the year 1940 (i.e., before the era of antibiotics) and had then been stored in a lyophilized form in sealed vials. The enterobacterial strains were originally collected from many different parts of the world, including Europe, the Middle East, Russia, and North America. Most of them were viable when the tubes were opened. The strain collection included 433 isolates, which were examined for antibiotic resistance genes and for conjugatable plasmid replicons. Regarding resistance, they were tested for some 10 different antibiotics, which are used clinically today. Only two resistance traits were found, and neither was transferable in conjugation experiments. Of the 30 strains of *Klebsiella* in the collection, only one showed resistance to ampicillin, which was shown to be mediated by a chromosomal betalactamase known to be normally present in that particular *Klebsiella* biotype, *Friedländer's bacillus*, which was found in the collection. The other resistance trait found in the collection was tetracycline resistance. It was observed in nine of the 16 *Proteus* strains identified in the collection of 433 isolates. Tetracycline resistance located on the chromosome is found as a normal *Proteus* trait. All 433 isolates were also examined for the occurrence of conjugatable plasmids. This was performed with the help of the mobilization phenomenon, described earlier in the chapter. That is, they were tested for their ability to transfer a small well-characterized but in itself nonconjugatable plasmid to a well-defined recipient by a triple cross. Three bacterial strains are involved. The first is the one tested for harboring a conjugatable plasmid; the second carries the small, well-known, and nonconjugatable plasmid; and the third is a recipient that can be identified by selection markers.

By selection markers on the small plasmid (streptomycin or ampicillin resistance) and on the recipient, Naomi Datta and her co-workers could demonstrate that 104 of the 433 isolates of the strain collection actually possessed conjugatability; that is, they harbored plasmids carrying the conjugation mechanism described earlier. These isolates were collected in the period 1917–1941, that is, before antibiotics came into general use. The sizes of these plasmids were in the range 37.5 to 157.5 kb, as determined by gel electrophoresis. These sizes are comparable with those seen today for R plasmids. These old plasmids did not carry any resistance genes, however. Further investigations also showed that those plasmids were of the same *inc* types (see earlier in the chapter) as those we see among R plasmids today. The important interpretation of these results is that conjugatable plasmids were as common among enterobacteria before the antibiotics era as they are today. Resistance genes that are seen on conjugatable plasmids today, and which are spread horizontally very efficiently by these plasmids, have been taken up by genetic mechanisms under the selection pressure of heavy antibiotics distribution. A definition of these mechanisms then becomes very important for an understanding of resistance development.

TRANSPOSONS

By the localization on movable plasmids, resistance genes have access to utterly efficient vehicles for spreading in bacterial pop-ulations. The localization of resistance genes on plasmids is, in turn, dependent on being carried by transposons that could locate in plasmids by recombination. Bacterial transposons were originally observed in the laboratory of Naomi Datta, "the Grand Lady of R plasmids." In compatibility tests with two R plasmids, when a recombinant plasmid was introduced into the same strain of *E. coli*, the ampicillin resistance gene of one plasmid seemed to have jumped onto the other plasmid. More extensive studies of this phenomenon later led to the proposition of transposons in bacteria. Transposons are extrachromosomal genetic elements, which, however, cannot live an independent life, in the sense that unlike plasmids, they do not have the ability to replicate on their own. They must rely on other genetic elements by being borne on them and replicate with them. Transposons have the ability to move from plasmid to plasmid, or from plasmid to chromosome, or from chromosome to plasmid, and since they can carry antibiotic resistance genes, transposons and transposition form another level of the spread of antibiotic resistance. That parts of the genome could move between different localizations within the genome was known as early as the 1950s. However, precise observations at the molecular level regarding transposons, as the defined genetic elements were called, were not made until the 1970s. The initial observations were about gene mutations, which were not caused by base changes but by DNA fragments that had moved into the gene, inactivating it. The same DNA fragment could be cut out to restore the function of the gene. These DNA fragments that showed spontaneous movability within the genome, denoted *insertion sequences* (ISs), turned out to be relatively short, about 2000 base pairs (2 kb). The movability of these insertion sequences was shown to be connected to specified nucleotide sequences at their ends. The sizes of these ends were up to several tens of nucleotides and their sequences were palindromic; that is, they were invertedly repeated. The sequence at one end is identical to that of the other end but in the opposite direction. The movable IS fragment also contains a gene expressing a specific endonuclease, a DNA splitting enzyme, which in this context is denoted transposase and is involved in the movability process, the transposition. In addition to being mutagenic, the IS fragment has a much wider function, in that it can also carry other genes: for example, genes expressing antibiotic resistance. These resistance genes then become movable together with the IS fragment, and this genetic entity is then denoted Tn (for "transposon"; Fig. 10.4).

An example of this was described in Chapter 3, where resistance to trimethoprim mediated by *dfr9* was described as being

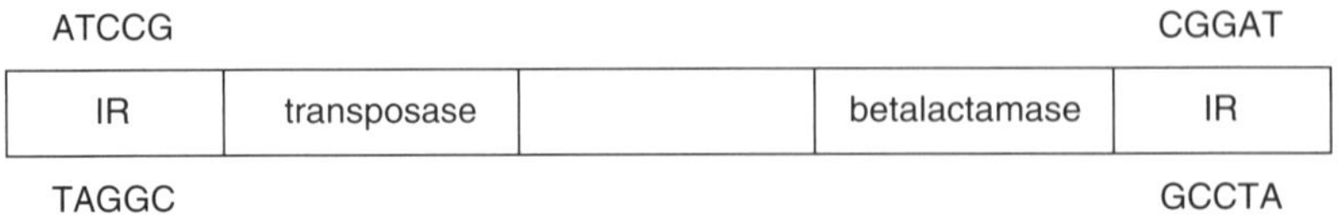

ATCCG CGGAT

IR	transposase		betalactamase	IR

TAGGC GCCTA

FIGURE 10.4 Schematic illustration of a transposon. The invertedly repeated end sequences mentioned in the text (IR, inverted repeat) are here represented by a randomly chosen five-base pair sequence. The IRs can vary largely in size between different transposons. The IRs are recognized by the transposase, which mediates the movability of the transposon. As mentioned in the text, transposons are important vehicles for the spread of antibiotics resistance, and as an illustration of this, a structural gene for betalactamase is represented here.

associated with the transposon Tn5393. Quite a few different transposons carrying different resistance genes are known. They are denoted by Tn and a number (e.g., Tn1546), described in Chapter 5 as carrying a set of genes together effecting vancomycin resistance in a host. The transposon with its transposition mechanism is, of course, a very efficient vehicle for the dissemination of antibiotic resistance, creating movability in different directions between bacterial chromosomes and bacterial plasmids.

The transposition proper can take place by two different genetic mechanisms. One of them, "cut and paste," is effected by the transposase simply cutting out the transposon from its original location, cutting up its recipient site, and placing the transposon at its new site on the recipient (Fig. 10.5). The second mechanism includes the replication of the transposon such that one copy of the transposon is left at its original site while one copy is inserted into the recipient DNA. In the latter course of action, the donor element (e.g., a plasmid) forms a covalently bound structure with the recipient structure, which could also be a plasmid, and will then be included in a *cointegrate*, as it is called, a large circle comprising both plasmids (Fig. 10.6). The transposon-borne resolvase enzyme will finally resolve the

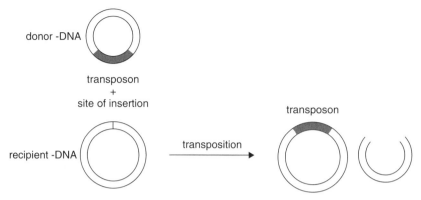

FIGURE 10.5 Representation of transposition. The simplest mechanism of transposition from one circular DNA molecule to another. The transposon is cut out of its position in the donor DNA molecule by its own transposase to be inserted at the receptor position of another DNA molecule, also by its own transposase.

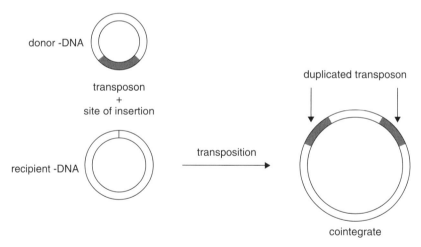

FIGURE 10.6 Schematic representation of replicative transposition. The transposon is replicated while the donor and the recipient are bound together. This will result in a cointegrate structure, where donor and recipient are linked together covalently. The donor and recipient will then resolve into the original donor plasmid, with the recipient plasmid now carrying a copy of the transposon.

cointegrate to re-form the two original DNA elements (plasmids), each now carrying a transposon.

INTEGRONS

In the hierarchy of elements disseminating antibiotic resistance genes such as transferable plasmids and transposons, there is still another level, the integron, which could carry several resistance genes. This genetic entity has no genetic movability of its own. It is stationary and is usually found incorporated into transposons. The integron can, however, give mobility to those resistance genes, which it harbors as movable cassettes, which makes it a natural genetic engineering platform. The cassette can be looked upon as a very efficient package for resistance genes in that the cassette structure mediates a genetic movability to single resistance genes, a powerful recombination machinery. The cassette has only two functional components; one is the structural resistance gene without a promoter, the other is a recombination component called 59*be* (base element). Despite its name, the latter can vary in size between 57 and 141 base pairs and is located downstream of the structural gene. The cassette can exist in two forms: either as a circular nonreplicating molecule, or integrated in the *att*I site of the integron (Fig. 10.7).

Cassette integration or excision is effected by an integrase, expressed from a gene *int* also located on the integron. The integrase catalyzes a site-specific recombination, which includes recognition of the 59*be* of the cassette by the integrase, which by recombination integrates it at the specific *att*I site located at the upstream end of the *int* gene. The 59be end of the integrated cassette forms a new specific recombination site, *att*C, which is recognized by the integrase, particularly at the cutting out of cassettes. It could be mentioned here that the 3' end of the *att*C has a constant sequence GTTRRRY (R = purin, Y = pyrimidine),

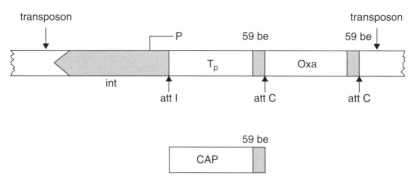

FIGURE 10.7 Schematic description of an integron. The integron is described here as being inserted in a transposon. The integrase gene *int* is expressed from right to left, while the resistance genes (in this case, *Tp* for trimethoprim resistance via drug-resistant dihydrofolate reductase, and *Oxa* for oxacillin resistance via oxacillin-degrading betalactamase) are expressed from left to right and from the promoter *P* located in the upstream part of the *int* gene. The *att*I and *att*C loci are the integrase recognition sites mentioned in the text. The lower part of the figure depicts a cassette with its 59*be* part and its structural gene, which in this case is *CAP*, representing chloramphenicol acetyl transferase mediating resistance to chloramphenicol.

which is called the *core site*, which then, in effect, will flank all the cassettes inserted in the integron. It should be added that there is an inverse core site (RYYYAAC) at the 5' end of the *att*C, corresponding to the 59*be* element. These characteristics are involved in the integrase recognition mechanism. Further cassettes can be inserted at the *att*I site, giving the integron the ability to form an assortment of integron-borne combinations of antibiotic resistance genes. A single integron has been observed to carry eight different antibiotic resistance cassettes. The integrase of the integron can, correspondingly, cut out cassettes. This means that integron cassettes are quite mobile (Fig. 10.7).

As mentioned, the cassette does not include a promoter for the gene it carries. But in the upstream end of the *int* gene bordering on the first cassette there is a strong promoter working in the direction opposite to the *int* gene transcription (Fig. 10.7). This promoter is responsible for the transcription of the structural genes in all the cassettes situated downstream of the *att*I site. The integron is thus a very efficient vehicle for the spread of resistance genes. It can do this with only five genetic components: one gene *int* expressing integrase, one DNA site *att*I recognized by the integrase, one promoter for the expression of the cassette-borne genes, and the two cassette components, a structural gene and 59*be*. More than five different types of antibiotic resistance–carrying integrons have now been described. They differ among themselves by different amino acid sequences of their integrase enzymes. Hundreds of different integron-borne resistance gene cassettes have been identified. They differ by carrying different resistance genes against many different antibiotics, and also by differences in the nucleotide sequence of the 59*be*. The different cassettes do not seem to have a specificity for a particular integrase. The same cassette can be found in different integrons with different integrases. Integrons can move from host to host borne on transposons. They carry a mobile genetic repertoire, the units of which efficiently move from integron to integron and then contribute intensively to the spread of resistance genes.

Antibacterial agents, antibiotics, have been distributed in the biosphere for about 70 years. From an evolutionary point of view, this is a very short period of time, and the degree of homology between the five integrases is roughly 40 to 60%, suggesting that their evolutionary divergence extends much longer. The integron cannot be thought of as having developed during this time. A similar structure must have been available in the microbial world for a long time, which later, under the selection pressure of antibiotics, developed into the resistance-spreading genetic vehicle we see today. Such ancestral structures have actually been observed. In the chromosomal genome of the cholera bacillus,

Vibrio cholerae, for example, a genetic structure has been found that was given the name *superintegron*. This consists of a group of genes in which the individual genes are separated by short nucleotide sequences of 123 to 126 base pairs, called VCRs. These short sequences are very similar to 59*be*, described as a cassette component of the resistance-mediating integrons.

In several cases that were analyzed, they are actually identical. One case is a resistance cassette carrying trimethoprim resistance (*dfr*6), and another is that of a betalactam resistance cassette carrying the gene *carb*4. The superintegron structure has also been observed in other bacterial species. It could be surmised to be an old structure evolutionarily, which by being able to exchange genes, has given its host a valuable adaptability upon the advent of drastic changes in the environment. In the case of the cholera bacillus, it is known that it survives bound to plankton in the sea, and then appears at times as a pathogen in epidemics. Most of the cassette-borne genes in the superintegrons studied are unknown and have no counterparts in available databases. Furthermore, the cassettes in superintegrons can be quite numerous. In the case of the epidemiologically well-known *Vibrio cholerae* strain El Tor, the superintegron found carries an array of 179 cassettes, occupying about 3% of the total genome. In a similar fashion, the antibiotic resistance integron mediates adaptability and survival following the drastic environmental changes that the distribution of antibiotics has created. Speculatively, resistance integrons could have emerged from superintegrons by genetic recombinations under the selection pressure of antibiotics, by the entrapment of integrase genes and their corresponding *att*I sites by mobile genetic structures such as transposons. Thus by use of plasmid replicons, recombination mechanisms, and gene transfer mechanisms, bacteria can use the enormous pool of antibiotic resistance genes that are accessible when needed.

Finally, it may be concluded that bacteria are survivors and that whatever antimicrobial agent is introduced into clinical practise, bacteria will survive and thrive. No microbiologist can refrain from marveling at the ability of microbes to resist our best efforts to control or eliminate them. They have inhabited the world and adapted to many hostile environments for almost 4 billion years, so we cannot believe that we can conquer them within some seven decades of remedial effort.

CHAPTER 11

HOW TO MANAGE ANTIBIOTIC RESISTANCE

Antibiotics have a unique position among medicines in that they act against foreign cells, bacteria, which can grow independently in human tissues, which offer good nutrient conditions for bacterial growth. Pathogenic bacteria growing in human tissues have many different receptors for selective antibiotic action. Medicines that act pharmacologically, on the other hand, interfere with unchangeable physiological receptors in the tissue cells of humans and animals. For bacteria the presence of antibiotics involves a dramatic change in the environment, and the great ability of bacteria to adapt to changes in the environment (e.g., by mutations) is in large part dependent on their rapid growth. This rate of growth is reflected in very short generation times, which in the test tube can be measured in minutes and in human tissues in hours.

Antibiotics and Antibiotics Resistance, First Edition. Ola Sköld.
© 2011 John Wiley & Sons, Inc. Published 2011 by John Wiley & Sons, Inc.

CROSS RESISTANCE BETWEEN RELATED ANTIBIOTICS

The impression that a great many antibiotics are available is misleading from a resistance point of view. Available antibiotics are in many cases related to each other in terms of mechanisms of action on bacteria and then encounter similar mechanisms of resistance in bacteria. Antibiotics can be seen as appearing in families within which cross resistance is common. In lists of antibacterial agents used for medical purposes in Western industrialized countries, there are ususally about 60 of these agents, antibiotics for systemic use. Roughly 50 of these can be included in five families, within which cross resistance occurs. The largest of these families is that of the betalactams, comprising about 30 members, including penicillins, cefalosporins, and monobactams. Cross resistance within this group is caused by resistance-mediating betalactamases, which can often hydrolyze the betalactam ring of many members of the betalactam group to inctivate their antibacterial action, and as described in Chapter 4, the betalactamases can change mutationally to adapt to different betalactams under the selection pressure of newly introduced betalactam derivatives (extended spectrum betalactamases). Other antibiotics families are tetracyclines usually with about four members; aminoglycosides with some four members; quinolones with perhaps five members; and macrolides, including lincosamides and streptogramins, comprising almost 10 members. Within all these antibiotic groups there is cross resistance.

THE EVOLUTION OF ANTIBACTERIAL RESISTANCE

The bacterial adaptation to antibiotics by developing resistance can be looked upon as Darwinian evolution that has taken place and is taking place right now, since the beginning of the antibiotics era. No microbiologist can avoid admiring the great number of often complicated genetic mechanisms that this evolution has been able to find and develop to protect bacteria from those industrially produced environmental toxins that antibiotics are in the microbial world. A good example is the integron mechanism, described in Chapter 10, where evolution, under the selection pressure of antibiotics, has been able to adapt an ancient gene transport mechanism into a very efficient tool for the dissemination of antibiotic resistance genes among bacteria. With an anthropomorphic perspective, medicinal chemists trying to produce new antibacterial agents can look at the bacterial world as a very old and wise antagonist. Human intelligence and ingenuity are measured against the genes of bacteria. Plasmid-borne quinolone resistance is an illustration of this. For decades, molecular biologists and microbiologists were certain that on the basis of what was known of the chemical properties of quinolones, and of the structure and function of DNA gyrase, this type of quinolone resistance could not exist. Still it was observed and its mechanism characterized a few years ago. This mechanism was completely unexpected and of a type previously unknown. Studies of this mechanism have actually led to basic studies regarding a new aspect of DNA replication (Chapter 9).

The development and evolution of antibiotic resistance can be looked upon as a modern and very rapidly unfolding example of the principles of Charles Darwin described in *The Origin of Species*. The organisms against which antibiotics direct their action grow very fast and are subjected to spontaneous muta-tions. By the mechanisms of horizontal movement of genes and of recombination, they also have access to a wide variety of genes from a very large group of environmental microorganisms. All these mechanisms and properties, at a low frequency, give rise to single resistant organisms, which then possess an acute sur-vival ability in the environmental niche formed by the presence of antibacterial agents, and will be selected to grow. This niche is humanmade, and the present situation regarding antibiotic resistance can be seen as having been formed in the interplay between humans and microorganisms.

HOW TO COUNTERACT RESISTANCE DEVELOPMENT

Antibiotics have given us a health standard that we tend to take for granted. This standard is threatened by resistance development, which is certainly very slow, but will in the long run interfere severely with the possibility of treating bacterial infections. Examples of acute situations in which all available antibiotics have been without effect because of resistance have been described internationally.

Four basic principles for mastering antibiotic resistance could be discerned. The first is simply to try to curtail the use of antibiotics by using them more specifically via strict bacterial diagnosis and resistance determinations. The intension here is to lower the selection pressure, to at least slow down the development of resistance. The second principle is to investigate the origin of resistance and its dissemination in order to find ways to neutralize its effects. The third principle includes making an inventory of antibacterial agents that have been left on the shelf by the pharmaceutical industry, possibly because of a certain level of observed toxicity. In the end we might have to chose between the possibility of treating serious infections and the risk of side effects from the use of antibiotics. The fourth and most important basic principle for mastering antibiotic resistance is to try to find genuinely new antibacterial agents. The pharmaceutical industry has shown a diminishing interest in this area for several years, however, at least regarding the continuation of the old tradition of screening for natural products. This is understandable. If the agent is efficient, the infection heals quickly and medication can stop. The sales are relatively small. Also, as has been described, resistance appears rather soon after introduction of the new agent. Antibiotics are therefore not that interesting from a sales point of view.

Curtailing the Use of Antibiotics

In the discussion of counteracting or at least slowing down resistance development by curbing the use of antibiotics, it becomes relevant to ask if the resistance properties of bacteria are reversible. That is, will antibiotic susceptibility return if the selection pressure ceases? If this is the case, it invites a solution that would include a cyclic use of antibiotics. That is, when high and widely spread resistance strikes one antibiotic, its distribution is stopped and it is exchanged for another until susceptibility possibly returns through evolutionary development. It is logical to surmise that resistance involves a biological cost to the bacterium, because it includes a molecular deviation from the normal physiology of the bacterial cell, which has adapted to its environment for a long period during evolution.

That this is a valid argument can easily be shown experimentally. Spontaneous test tube mutants resistant against sulfonamides, for example, show that they have had to pay a price for their resistance. The mutation hits the sulfonamide target enzyme, dihydropteroate synthase, which then shows a lower susceptibility to sulfonamides but also makes the enzyme require a higher concentration of its normal substrate (p-aminobenzoic acid) for optimal function. The resistant bacterium has traded off part of its general survival value for the acutely necessary resistance in the presence of sulfonamide. It has also been shown experimentally that in a mixture of susceptible and resistant bacteria that are resistant either by mutation or by plasmid-borne resistance genes, resistance is a strain on bacterial growth, in that susceptible bacteria will soon dominate in a culture grown in the absence of antibiotic.

In line with this thinking, there was an interesting clinical experiment in southern Sweden, where outpatient doctors in a one-county area decided not to prescribe trimethoprim for bacterial infections, for which equivalent antibacterial agents were available. The purpose was to discover if the increasing trimethoprim resistance that had been observed in the area would stabilize or possibly diminish. The results were negative, however, probably because plasmids carrying trimethoprim resistance also carry other resistance genes, and trimethoprim resistance is then co-selected with them.

Resistance evolution is very efficient in a clinical context. This was illustrated in Chapter 3, where we discussed sulfonamide resistance in *Neisseria meningitidis*. This bacterium seems to have the ability to neutralize the growth strain of resistance by the introduction of compensating mutations. This could be compared to the argument in an earlier section, where experimental results showed sulfonamide resistance mutations to have a price in the form of an increased K_m value for the normal substrate of the target enzyme mutated. Normal K_m values are, however, seen in sulfonamide-resistant clinical isolates of *N. meningitidis*. This must mean that other mutations in the gene for the target enzyme dihydropteroate synthase have changed the conformation of the enzyme to normalize substrate binding. This is an evolutionary phenomenon leading to the complete bacterial adaptation to the presence of sulfonamides. Importantly, this also means that the resistance is irreversible. This is corroborated by the fact that sulfonamide-resistant strains of *N. meningitidis* are continuously isolated from clinical specimens, despite the fact that for decades, sulfonamides have not been used systemically for the treatment of these bacteria. This argument is very important when judging the future of antibacterial agents.

One area of obvious restriction in the distribution of antibiotics is their use for growth promotion in animal husbandry.

This was suggested with great foresight in 1969 by a report presented to the British government by a committee chaired by M. M. Swann. It took almost 40 years, however, for these ideas to be translated into legislation in Europe. In the United States, rules in this area are still awaiting realization.

Introduction of Truly New Antibacterial Agents

A solution to the present clinical situation with increasing antibiotic resistance would be to find new antibacterial agents with truly new properties of action. Literally thousands of antibiotics have been isolated since the 1940s, but only a small fraction of these have proved suitable for medical and veterinary use. Also, the pace of discovering new antibacterial agents has slowed through the years. Trimethoprim was introduced in 1970 and oxazolidinones in 2000, both representing new antibacterial agents in the true sense at their introduction, that is, no truly new antibacterials were introduced for 30 years. This could be taken to mean that the screening of natural products and of presumed antimetabolites will be able to contribute less and less to finding new antibiotics. New principles for antibacterial treatment that are conceptually different from the antibiotics used presently are needed urgently. Agents of this type can be discerned. Two examples follow. Another example demonstrating the difficulties in this approach is also described.

Antibacterial Peptides

Humans and animals have an inborn mechanism of protection against bacterial infections which acts instantly; that is, it works differently from the immune system, the response of which has to await the growth of antibody-producing cells. Inborn immunity, or innate immunity as it has been called, works by means of a sort of peptide antibiotic produced by the tissue cells and comprising a sort of first defense against bacterial infection. Host defense peptides or antibacterial peptides of this type seem to be produced by all multicellular organisms, including plants, and also by many unicellular organisms. Compared to antibiotics, which are target-specific molecules acting in a single well-defined manner, these peptides have more complex inhibitory patterns and multiple activities. They are amphiphile, cationic molecules, which with their positive charge bind to the negatively charged membrane of microbes. The crucial physicochemical feature for the antibiotic activity of host defense peptides is their amphiphilic character, which enables them to adopt conformations in which polar and charged amino acid side chains orient to one side and apolar residues to the other (Fig. 11.1). These peptides can then bind to negatively charged bacterial surfaces and integrate into and disrupt underlying cytoplasmic membranes. There is substantial evidence that the charge-mediated binding of host defense peptides is critical for their antibacterial activity.

This knowledge regarding the lipid bilayer disturbing effect is, however, based on studies of model membranes, which leaves many questions regarding the precise mechanism of the bacteria-killing activity. Others also work by different mechanisms. Several hundred peptides of this kind have now been described and classified according to structural characteristics; they include alpha- and beta-defensins, cathelicidines, cecropins, magainins, bactenecins, and protegrins. Those that are called cathelicidines and defensins dominate within the group of vertebrates. Cathelicidines in an active form vary in size between 12 and about 80 amino acid residues and appear in various tertiary structures. Defensins are more similar between themselves and form a group of small cysteine-rich peptides whose tertiary structures are stabilized by three or four intramolecular cystine

β-Defensin
Human hBD3

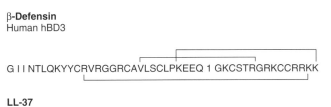

G I I NTLQKYYCRVRGGRCAVLSCLPKEEQ 1 GKCSTRGRKCCRRKK

LL-37
Human cathelicidin

LLGDFFRKSKEKIGKEFKRIVQRIKDFLRNLVPRTES

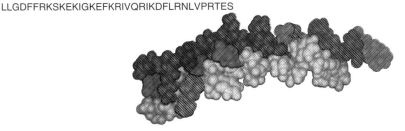

FIGURE 11.1 Antibacterial peptides. Schematic description of a betade-fensin (human hBD3) and of a cathelicidin (human LL-37). Amino acid sequences are given for the two peptides and for the human betade-fensin, also the intramolecular cystine disulfide bridges mentioned in the text. The pronounced amphiphilicity of LL-37 is demonstrated in the spatial structure, with hydrophobic residues in light gray at the bottom of the molecule pictured, negatively charged side chains in darker gray at five locations in the molecule depicted, and positively charged residues in black, mainly at the upper part of the depicted molecule.

disulfide bridges. Defensins and other antimicrobial peptides are possible candidates to be pharmaceutical preparations for use in the clinical treatment of bacterial infections.

A rather recently published example of such a candidate peptide is plectasin, an antimicrobial defensin isolated from the mold *Pseudoplectania nigrella*. It was reported that the plectasin-producing gene could be transferred to another fungus, which could produce and excrete plectasin in large amounts. This could be a solution to a serious problem with antibacterial peptides, which is to produce them in sufficient amounts and in a way that is economically defendable. Determinations in vitro showed plectasin to have a bactericidal effect against several species of gram-positive bacteria, such as *Streptococcus pneumoniae*. The bactericidal efficiency was comparable to that of penicillin and vancomycin. In animal experiments with experimental peritonitis in mice caused by *S. pneumoniae*, intravenously administered plectasin showed a survival effect. Plectasin is also effective against streptococci, and a modified derivative of it is effective against staphylococci, including MRSA. The mice test is a parallel to the historically famous experiment with penicillin by Howard Florey in May 1940. There is more to this parallel than was originally thought, however. In a recent report it was found, astonishingly, that the plectasin peptide of 40 amino acid residues with its amphipathic nature does not compromise bacterial membrane integrity as do similar defensins with the characteristic intramolecular cystine disulfide bridges stabilizing their tertiary structures. Instead, it was actually found to interfere with bacterial cell wall synthesis, which was originally observed as severe cell-shaped deformations occurring in its presence.

In more detail, the action of plectasin was more like the glycopeptide antibiotics (such as vancomycin, Chapter 5) found to form a stoichiometric complex with an intermediate in the biosynthetic pathway of cell wall formation. This intermediate is the glycopeptide–lipid complex, which translocates across the cytoplasmic membrane to the outside, where the glycopeptide is incorporated into the peptidoglycan polymer through the activity of transglycosylases and transpeptidases (see Chapter 4). There is no cross resistance between vancomycin and plectasin. It can be concluded that plectasin is a promising substance for further drug development. The results obtained seem to show that in the future, antibacterial peptides could play an important role in the treatment of infectious disease. One obstacle is that they are peptides susceptible to degradation in the gastrointestinal tract.

Inhibition of Pathogenicity

Another example of a completely new approach to the treatment of bacterial infections is to try to interfere with the pathogenicity of the infecting bacteria with medicines. This could, for example, be to inhibit the adhesion of bacteria to the epithelial cells of the ureters in the urinary tract in severe infections in the upper parts of this tract. Another approach of the same type, presently under development, is related to the secretion system of type III, which in many pathogenic gram-negative bacteria is decisive for virulence and pathogenicity. Pathogenic bacteria such as *Shigella* and *Salmonella* use this type III system to deliver toxins into the cells of the organism infected. The excretion system of type III can be looked upon as a syringe which is able to perforate human intestinal cells, for example, and inject toxins and other pathogenic substances into them. It then becomes a very important part of bacterial pathogenicicty. The secretion system of type III has a complicated structure consisting of several tens of bacterial proteins. This complexity and the fact that transport through the syringe needle requires energy makes it likely that the proper secretion mechanism could be inhibited without interfering with the growth of the bacterium. Small molecular inhibitors with this effect have been identified and ought to be developed into anti-infectious remedies. The new and important aspect of this approach is that only the pathogenicity is interfered with; bacterial growth and survival are unaffected. This is different from other antibacterial agents and eliminates the immediate risk of resistance development. Bacterial growth is normal, which means that mutations affecting the pathogenicity inhibition are not selected. Anthropomorphically, it could be expressed as if the bacterium does not know about being exposed to an inhibiting agent, because the survival value of its pathogenicity probably works only over a very long perspective of time.

Inhibition of Bacterial Fatty Acid Synthesis

Pharmaceutical companies have to a large extent retreated from the field of antibacterial drugs, concentrating instead on chronic diseases, which has market advantages. Earlier, there was a cooperation between the health care and pharmaceutical industries, which has now ceased, particularly regarding antibacterial agents. It was therefore very encouraging that the Merck pharmaceutical company took on the work of characterizing and developing a new approach to antibacterial action. As it turned out, it also became a good illustration of the great risks involved with developing a new antibacterial agent. This particular approach began with a report about a new antibiotic produced by the soil bacterium *Streptomyces platensis* isolated from a soil sample from South Africa. The finding was the result of a large screening program involving 250,000 extracts from drug-producing microorganisms. The antibiotic derived from *S. platensis* was named *platensimycin*. It turned out to be a small molecule (molecular mass: 441 Da), consisting of two distinct structural elements: 3-amino-2,4-dihydroxybenzoic acid and lipophilic pentacyclic ketolide, linked together by an amide bond. Platensimycin showed a new mechanism of action, interfering selectively with the enzymatic elongation mechanism at the bacterial synthesis of fatty acids, which in sizes of 8 to 18 carbon atoms build bacterial membranes and cell surfaces. It ought to be pointed out here that inhibition of bacterial fatty acid synthesis for antibacterial action was used before in the action of the tuberculostatic agent of isoniazid, discussed in Chapter 9. Isoniazid activated to isonicotinic acid inside the tuberculosis bacterium inhibits the formation of mycolic acids, which are essential fatty acid components of the bacterial cell wall in

M. tuberculosis. So far, platensimycin has only been tested in vitro and in preliminary animal experiments with mice, where it showed inhibiting effects against staphylococci and pneumococci similar to those of penicillin against susceptible strains of these bacteria. There is still a long way to a clinically useful agent, and there would be a risk of resistance by mutational enzyme changes. Again it is interesting that the extensive research work regarding platensimycin was performed and the cost defrayed by a large pharmaceutical company, which by economic considerations seems to continue research regarding antibacterial agents.

To explain the scarcity of new antibacterial agents and the risks involved in their development, the future potential of platensimycin is important to assess. The future use of platensimycin as an antibiotic was hit by a great disappointment. The biosynthetic machinery of fatty acid formation is encoded by several bacterial genes involving the *fab* loci of the bacterial genome. Fab proteins come together to construct fatty acids two carbon atoms at a time in a cyclic process. This biosynthetic pathway is essential for the formation of cellular membranes in many bacterial pathogens. The process is distinct from fatty acid biosynthesis in mammalian cells, which suggests that its inhibition in bacteria could be selective. Yet older studies, from the 1970s, showed that bacteria could acquire fatty acids from their surroundings and incorporate them into their cell membranes. In a recent report, evidence was presented to question antibiotic therapies that target fatty acid biosynthesis. Inhibitors of fatty acid synthesis were quite effective at inhibiting the growth of pathogenic strains resistant to other antibiotics in standard laboratory media (which lack fatty acids), but this effect was abolished when fatty acids were added or when human serum, which is rich in fatty acids, was added. Moreover, the report presented experiments with mutant strains of bacteria lacking many of the *fab* genes, which would flourish in the fatty acid–rich human serum. These observations would raise the bar for target validation not only for platensimycin but for future drug discovery in general.

RESISTANCE DEVELOPMENT ACCELERATES

A newly published report from a Canadian laboratory for the study of antibiotics makes it clear that in many ways we are in a hurry to develop new antibacterial agents. The authors of this report define what they call the *resistome*, comprising a gigantic collection of antibiotic resistance genes among soil-living microorganisms. This concept of the resistome will dramatically reshape our approach to finding new antibacterial drugs. There is abundant information regarding soil bacteria producing and encountering large amounts of antibiotics, which has meant that these organisms have evolved corresponding sensing and evading strategies. It is a fact that most clinically relevant antibiotics originate from soil-dwelling actinomycetes. Antibiotic producers harbor resistance elements for self-protection, which are often found together with antibiotic biosynthetic operons. Genes ortologous to these have been observed on mobile genetic elements in resistant pathogenic bacteria isolated from patients.

For example, and as mentioned earlier, aminoglycoside-modifying enzymes (Chapter 6) and the lactate-substituting machinery making the peptidoglycan synthesis insensitive to vancomycin probably originated in soil-dwelling antibiotic producers (Chapter 5). The presence of antibiotics in the environment has been shown to promote the acquisition or independent evolution of specific resistance elements in soil organisms in the absence of innate antibiotic production. The soil could thus be looked at as a large reservoir for resistance, the largest part of which might not yet have emerged in clinically important bacteria. Consequently, an understanding of the soil resistome (i.e., identification of resistance determinants in the resistome) could serve as an early warning system for the occurrence of new resistance mechanisms that may emerge as clinical problems. The report mentioned is a systematic study of 480 morphologically different soil microbes regarding their resistance to 21 different antibacterial agents, including natural products such as vancomycin and erythromycin, and also completely synthetic molecules such as quinolones, sulfonamides, trimethoprim, and linezolid. Many of the agents tested were well established, but importantly, antibacterial drugs that have only recently been approved for clinical use were also tested. Astonishingly, every isolate was found to be multidrug resistant to seven or eight antibiotics on average, with two strains being resistant to 15 of the 21 antibacterial agents tested. Interestingly, five of the vancomycin-resistant soil microbe isolates were, by the use of polymerase chain reaction, shown to carry the cluster of three genes that in clinical isolates of vancomycin-resistant pathogenic bacteria has been shown to mediate resistance to this drug. Regarding the completely synthetic fluoroquinolones, clinical resistance occurs primarily through point mutations in the bacterial target enzyme, DNA gyrase. Despite the lack of known prior exposure to fluoroquinolones, some 10% of the soil microbes in the study demonstrated intrinsic resistance to ciprofloxacin.

A closer investigation of the quinolone resistance–determining region in these soil strains showed this to contain mutational amino acid substitutions at locations commonly associated with clinical ciprofloxacin resistance, but also at novel sites, including one with the highest MIC value. All the soil microbe strains were resistant to the synthetic agent trimethoprim, which as mentioned earlier, works by inhibiting the bacterial dihydrofolate reductase. The frequency of high-level resistance to many antibiotics used for decades as well as to those recently approved for human use indicates a remarkable potential for antibiotic resistance in soil organisms. Further studies along these lines could assist in the elucidation of new resistance mechanisms that may emerge clinically, as well as serve as a foundation for the development of new antibiotics. These results, combined with earlier experiences of the spread of antibiotics resistance by efficient gene transport mechanisms, indicate that resistance development is probably going to accelerate. The observations described could lead to the view that the wonderful asset of antibiotics has been available on loan from nature, and that this loan is now expiring slowly, with devalued assets. There is a threat of foreclosure.

INDEX

Antibiotics and Antibiotics Resistance, First Edition. Ola Sköld.
© 2011 John Wiley & Sons, Inc. Published 2011 by John Wiley & Sons, Inc.